THE DOCTORS WEIGHT LOSS DIET

YOUR MEDICALLY APPROVED
LOW-CARB SOLUTION FOR TOTAL HEALTH

AIMEE ARISTOTELOUS & RICHARD OLIVA

Foreword by Katherine Rodriguez, MD

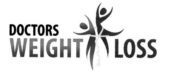

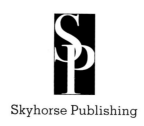

Skyhorse Publishing

Skyhorse Publishing books may be purchased in bulk at special discounts for sales promotion, corporate gifts, fund-raising, or educational purposes. Special editions can also be created to specifications. For details, contact the Special Sales Department, Skyhorse Publishing, 307 West 36th Street, 11th Floor, New York, NY 10018 or info@skyhorsepublishing.com.

Skyhorse® and Skyhorse Publishing® are registered trademarks of Skyhorse Publishing, Inc.®, a Delaware corporation.

Visit our website at www.skyhorsepublishing.com.

10 9 8 7 6 5 4 3 2 1

Library of Congress Cataloging-in-Publication Data

Names: Aristotelous, Aimee, author. | Oliva, Richard, author. | Rodriguez, Katherine, other. | Doctors Weight Loss (Miami, Florida), author.
Title: The doctors weight loss diet : your medically approved low-carb solution for total health / Aimee Aristotelous and Richard Oliva ; foreword by Katherine Rodriguez, MD. Doctor Weight Loss.
Description: New York, NY : Skyhorse Publishing, [2022] | Includes bibliographical references and index. |
Identifiers: LCCN 2021041605 (print) | LCCN 2021041606 (ebook) | ISBN 9781510768383 (hardcover) | ISBN 9781510768390 (ebook)
Subjects: LCSH: Low-carbohydrate diet. | Weight loss.
Classification: LCC RM237.73 .A75 2022 (print) | LCC RM237.73 (ebook) | DDC 613.2/83--dc23
LC record available at https://lccn.loc.gov/2021041605
LC ebook record available at https://lccn.loc.gov/2021041606

Cover design by Sada Hudson and David Ter-Avanesyan
Cover images by Giovanni Paraison
All product images by Giovanni Paraison
Edited by Leah Zarra

Print ISBN: 978-1-5107-6838-3
Ebook ISBN: 978-1-5107-6839-0

Printed in China

Dedicated to Val Manocchio, MD,
an accomplished physician, father, and friend.

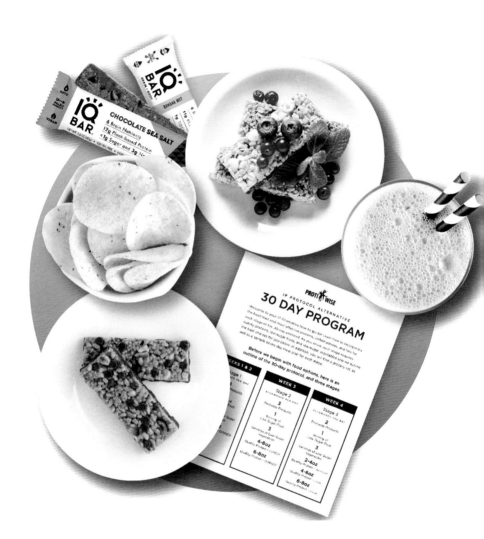

Contents

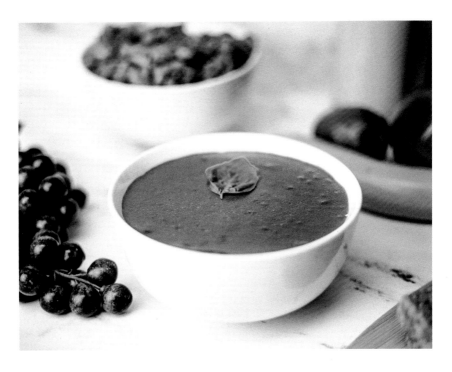

Foreword

BY KATHERINE RODRIGUEZ, MD

If you've ever struggled to lose weight or been a yo-yo dieter, this book is your solution. *The Doctors Weight Loss Diet* offers a unique shortcut to achieve your goals, which makes this plan far easier than most others. This medically approved protocol is low in sugar and carbohydrates, but the difference is you still get to cheat . . . on a daily basis.

As a medical doctor, I have been recommending a low-carbohydrate and high-protein nutrition plan to my patients for years. Numerous studies have documented the benefits of a low-sugar diet, citing positive health outcomes such as weight loss, decreased visceral fat, blood sugar stabilization, and calorie reduction. It can't be argued that a low-carbohydrate nutrition plan is one of the primary ways in which people lose weight and improve their health, so why isn't everyone employing this way of life? Simply put, it can be extremely difficult to give up carbohydrates, which in turn, means giving up sugar. This is how *The Doctors Weight Loss Diet* is different.

First of all, I'd like to clarify that this book instructs on everything that is low-carbohydrate and high-protein, giving a plethora of options regarding how to approach this lifestyle for effective weight loss. While they are not required, *The Doctors Weight Loss Diet* will educate you on medical-grade weight loss products. These are prepackaged foods that include your old favorites such as pasta, chocolate, cookies, pancakes, and chips, but they are specially formulated to fit the protocol—high in protein and low in carbohydrates. For those who struggle with giving up these items, I highly recommend using these products to make a comfortable transition to the low-carbohydrate lifestyle. I have had many patients who find it much more realistic to reach their weight loss goals by integrating medical-grade weight loss products as they are already portioned for you and truly taste like cheat foods.

The goal of this book is to take you from a high-carbohydrate and high-sugar lifestyle, and gently transition you to one that employs anywhere from 25 to 95 grams of carbohydrates per day. You will find several options to help you achieve this—meal plans that use only standard groceries, meal plans that use medical-grade weight loss products, simple recipes, more intricate recipes (for those who like spending time in the kitchen), grocery lists, and strategies for success. While you can choose your own nutrition adventure with this book, the common denominator is something we all need, and that's less sugar. The best part is, you will be instructed on exactly what to eat to achieve your desired weight, and you don't even have to exercise!

CHAPTER 1
Why the Standard American Diet Is Making Us Overweight

An estimated 160 million Americans are either overweight or obese. Of these 160 million people, almost 75 percent of American males and over 60 percent of females fall into these overweight and obese categories. An added concern is that almost 30 percent of male and female adolescents under the age of twenty are also either overweight or obese—this figure has risen from 19 percent in 1980.[1] In addition, roughly 50 percent of all American adults have one or more chronic diseases, often related to poor nutrition. During a time of various medical breakthroughs and advancements, we must start questioning why our nation's health is on the decline. A driving factor of the dismal state of our wellbeing is the reality that after decades of adjustments and modifications to our dietary recommendations, we are still being told to eat the wrong things.

The USDA MyPlate has made some small improvements when compared to 1992's famous (and faulty) Food Pyramid which suggested eating six to eleven servings of high-glycemic grains per day, as well as

---

1   Ng, Marie, Tom Fleming, Margaret Robinson, Blake Thomson, Nicholas Graetz, and Christopher Margano. "Global, Regional, and National Prevalence of Overweight and Obesity in Children and Adults during 1980–2013: A Systematic Analysis for the Global Burden of Disease Study 2013." *The Lancet*. May 28, 2014. Accessed February 06, 2019. https://www.thelancet.com/journals/lancet/article/PIIS0140-6736(14)60460–8/fulltext.

very little fat, despite how beneficial healthy fats are. However, many of the dietary guidelines for Americans still reek of monetary interests as opposed to the interests of the health of our public. Below is an example day of food which meets the USDA MyPlate's dietary recommendations for a 2,000-calorie diet.

USDA MyPlate Daily Recommended Foods and Servings (2,000-calorie diet)

3 cups of nonfat or low-fat milk
2 pieces of bread
1 cup of cereal
1 cup of pasta
1 cup of orange juice
1 cup of sliced bananas
1 cup of sweet potatoes
1 cup of broccoli
½ cup of carrots
4 ounces of chicken
1 egg
1 tablespoon of peanut butter

One may look at these recommendations and nod at the fact that they seem "normal" for today's standards and yes, they are normal; however, they are extremely faulty and actually contribute to serious medical conditions that run rampant in today's population, such as excessive weight gain and type 2 diabetes. Let's take this recommended daily intake of food and break it down into macronutrients (carbohydrates, protein, fat), as well as sugar so we can get a better understanding of the implications of these suggested foods.

As you can see, this suggested example of one day of "healthy food" results in 108 grams of sugar, as well as an abundance of high-glycemic carbohydrates, many of which come from processed foods. To put it into perspective, this amount of sugar and carbohydrates is equivalent to eating almost eleven glazed donuts in one day! One may say that sugars from

Food	Carbohydrates	Protein	Fat	Sugar
Whole wheat bread (2 slices)	24g	8g	2g	4g
Whole-grain cereal (1 cup)	29g	3g	2g	7g
Whole wheat pasta (1 cup)	41g	7g	2g	2g
Baked sweet potato (1 cup)	41g	4g	0g	13g
Broccoli (1 cup)	9g	3g	0g	2g
Carrots (½ cup)	6g	0g	2g	2g
Sliced banana (1 cup)	34g	2g	0g	18g
Orange juice (1 cup)	26g	2g	0g	22g
Chicken (4 ounces)	0g	30g	4g	0g
1 egg	1g	6g	5g	0g
Peanut butter (1 tablespoon)	3g	4g	8g	2g
2% milk (3 cups)	36g	24g	15g	36g
TOTALS	**250g**	**93g**	**40g**	**108g**

the above-listed foods are different than refined sugar; unfortunately, your body is negatively affected by too much sugar, regardless of whether it is from a natural source or from a donut. Another possible argument is that these foods do offer a variety of nutritional benefits (unlike eleven glazed donuts), thus justifying the sugar and carbohydrate intake. We will explain in later chapters how to get twice the nutrients that this typical plan offers, while consuming less than half the sugar, and no high-glycemic, processed carbohydrates (your carbs will come from healthier sources)!

Why is it so important that we reduce sugar and high-glycemic carbohydrate intake? According to the Center for Disease Control, more than 30 million Americans (around 10 percent) are afflicted with diabetes and 90 to 95 percent of these people have type 2 diabetes, which is often caused by diets that include too much sugar. Type 2 diabetes is also on the rise in groups where it used to be uncommon, such as in children and adolescents.[2]

---

2 "Type 2 Diabetes." Centers for Disease Control and Prevention. August 15, 2018. Accessed February 16, 2019. https://www.cdc.gov/diabetes/basics/type2.html.

If you are unaware of how type 2 diabetes develops, your pancreas makes the hormone insulin, and insulin is the regulating component that lets blood sugar into the cells to be used for energy. In the presence of type 2 diabetes, the insulin cannot make the cells respond, which results in insulin resistance. The pancreas reacts by creating more insulin but will not be able to keep up, resulting in rising blood sugar, which then establishes an environment for prediabetes and type 2 diabetes. Blood sugar levels that are too high are associated with a plethora of health issues including, but not limited to, excessive weight gain, heart disease, kidney disease, and vision loss. Fortunately, millions of these blood sugar–related ailments can be prevented or even managed with proper nutrition. Unfortunately, the current USDA nutrition recommendations that are provided to the public may actually cause these conditions—not prevent them!

You may be wondering, *Why are we told, by trusted governmental sources, to eat these foods if they may lead us down a path of type 2 diabetes, weight gain, and heart disease?* The United States Department of Agriculture plays a heavy role in determining these recommendations and then these same guidelines are incorporated in nutrition education curriculum which is taught to nutritionists, as well as some doctors. Essentially, as opposed to being based on scientific research and evidence, these recommendations are influenced by food producers, manufacturers, and special interest groups. One of the USDA's largest priorities is to strengthen and support food, agriculture, and farming industries, so these guidelines may be disproportionately based on profit as opposed to the health of the general population.[3]

Every year, the food industry donates millions of dollars to politicians who are in charge of making decisions regarding food regulation. This results in the industry's ability to market foods that are laden with sugar, salt, calories, and unhealthy fats. For example, the United States

---

3   Nestle, M. "Food Lobbies, the Food Pyramid, and U.S. Nutrition Policy." NCBI. July 1, 1993. Accessed February 16, 2019. https://www.ncbi.nlm.nih.gov/pubmed/8375951.

Department of Health and Human Services, as well as the USDA, vetoed their own expert panel's suggestions to reduce processed meat and sugary beverage consumption in their 2015–2020 Dietary Guidelines, despite substantial evidence that those items are harmful to public health.[4] Through this orchestration of campaign funding and lobbying, the food industry has effectively squashed and avoided evidence-based guidelines and taxation. Therefore, the industry has been somewhat allowed to market, formulate, and sell foods that are proven to be detrimental to health when consumed in excess.

In addition to our own regulatory agencies, which should be protecting our health by providing accurate information regarding nutrition, we have product powerhouses such as Coca-Cola who have donated millions of dollars to researchers whose intentions are to downplay the effects of sugary beverages on weight gain. Of course, we may expect this sort of underhanded activity when it comes to a large corporation that is trying to market its products, but we don't necessarily expect it from Harvard scientists. Back in the 1960s, Harvard scientists were paid by the sugar industry to minimize the link between heart disease and sugar. They had to name a new supposed culprit to take sugar's place—and the scapegoat was fat.[5] Unfortunately this faulty, money-based science has been the foundation for a variety of nutrition guidelines throughout the past five decades and has led the masses down a path of falsehoods when considering sugar, carbohydrate, and fat intake in their daily nutrition regimens.

The Doctors Weight Loss Diet will help you transition to a lower-carbohydrate lifestyle and free yourself from sugar addiction, all while enjoying delicious foods that will fend off cravings. After seeing the advice that is offered through our governmental agencies, online, in several literary sources, and even in nutritionists' and doctors' offices, it's no

---

4 Gostin, Lawrence O. ""Big Food" Is Making America Sick." NCBI. September 13, 2013. Accessed March 7, 2019. https://www.ncbi.nlm.nih.gov/pmc/articles/PMC5020160/
5 Damle, S. G. "Smart Sugar? The Sugar Conspiracy." NCBI. July 24, 2017. Accessed March 7, 2019. https://www.ncbi.nlm.nih.gov/pmc/articles/PMC5551319/.

wonder that millions of people are suffering from diet-related conditions despite the fact that they are, most likely, following mainstream nutrition advice. In coming chapters, you will find progressive and unbiased nutrition information that will be sure to put you on the right track for weight loss, toning, and impeccable health.

CHAPTER 2
If You're Addicted to Sugar, You're Not Alone

There is a two-pronged culprit contributing to the deteriorating health of our country—one being excessive carbohydrate intake, and the other sugar addiction. The average American currently consumes 57 pounds of added sugar in one year, which is roughly 17 teaspoons per day. Compare this sugar intake to an average consumption of two pounds per year, two hundred years ago. Our bodies are simply not built to have the ability to synthesize the amount of sugar that is commonly used today, resulting in a surge of type 2 diabetes, heart disease, and nonalcoholic fatty liver disease.

You may be thinking it's extreme to state that the average person consumes the equivalent of three desserts per day. While candies, cakes, cookies, and ice cream are obvious examples of sugar culprits, sweeteners are also added to the majority of our packaged foods, fueling the sugar industry's ability to exceed 100 billion dollars in recent years.[6] The industry is so profitable they must defend and downplay the effects of sugar, as illustrated by statements on their own website such as, "Sugar is simple, amazingly functional, and it's part of a balanced diet."[7] And yes, sugar can be consumed in true moderation but when you have a 100-billion

---

6   Dewan, S. "Global Markets for Sugars and Sweeteners in Processed Foods and Beverages." BCC Research, June 2015.
7   "Sugar & The Diet." The Sugar Association. Accessed March 5, 2020. https://www .sugar.org/diet/.

dollar industry whose primary interest is profits, our food supply ends up being plagued with a highly unbalanced proportion of sweetened products, making it virtually impossible to escape its presence. It's no surprise our society's health is on the decline when this money-fueled product is the primary culprit for a host of preventable diseases, and since sugar triggers the same responses in the body as some narcotics, it puts us at high risk for long-term addiction.[8]

To give you more clarity about how big this sugar business is, manufacturers add sugar to 74 percent of all of our packaged foods.[9] So even if you tend to skip the traditional dessert foods, you are still (likely) getting far more than the recommended daily intake. As an added concern, our society labels many of these sugar-laden foods as "healthy," which leads the masses down a path of weight gain and sugar-related diseases. How many times have you seen the "heart-healthy" selections on a restaurant menu or the "fit breakfast" at a hotel? Let's examine one of these typical meals, which many of us choose in an attempt to start the day off on the right foot.

Heart-Healthy Fit Breakfast Menu

Small plain croissant
Small yogurt parfait with fruit and granola
Orange juice

Heart-healthy breakfasts are typically classified by one characteristic: Being low in fat, meaning less than three grams of fat per 100 calories. No other considerations are taken into account, so we end up with recommended "healthy" fare that has exponential amounts of sugar, and that sugar, if not burned, will turn into fat. Let's break down this breakfast in terms of all macronutrients and sugars.

---

8 Avena, N., P. Rada, and B. Hoebel. "Evidence for Sugar Addiction: Behavioral and Neurochemical Effects of Intermittent, Excessive Sugar Intake." NCBI. *Neuroscience and Biobehavioral Reviews*, January 2008. https://www.ncbi.nlm.nih.gov/pmc/articles/PMC2235907/.

9 Ng, S. W., Slining, M. M., & Popkin, B. M. (2012). Use of caloric and noncaloric sweeteners in US consumer packaged foods, 2005–2009. *Journal of the Academy of Nutrition and Dietetics*, 112(11), 1828–1834.

Food	Calories	Fat	Carbohydrates	Protein	Sugar
1 croissant	170	6g	19g	3g	5g
1 parfait	210	3g	40g	6g	28g
1 cup orange juice	110	0g	26g	2g	22g
Total	**490**	**9g**	**85g**	**11g**	**55g**

This one 490-calorie breakfast is packed with 55 grams of sugar, which far exceeds the daily recommended intake of 37 grams of added sugar per day for men and 25 for women. The concern is the majority of people would think this is a healthy choice due to the fact that it is low in fat and devoid of items such as butter and egg yolks. Now add in food and beverages for the remainder of the day, and you can easily see how we are consuming several pounds of sugar per year.

When we as a society classify unhealthy sugar-laden meals like this as a good choice, it's no wonder people are confused about what to eat for weight loss and optimal wellness. Seventy-four percent of our packaged foods have added sugars, and because the Food and Drug Administration does not regulate terms such as "natural," "superfood," or "premium," we may falsely perceive many of these processed foods as conducive to weight loss and health. Several variations of the following supposed health food items tend to have the highest amounts of sugars despite the fact they are usually touted as being healthy, so it is important to always check the label for nutrition information, ingredients, and sugar content.

Flavored Yogurts

Some yogurts can be incorporated into your low-carb plan, but you must have a good look at the nutrition and ingredients label to ensure you're not packing in the same amount of sugar (or sometimes more) as you would with a bowl of ice cream. Flavored and low- or nonfat yogurts tend to be the biggest offenders, with upward of 47 grams of sugar per cup, which exceeds the limit of daily sugar intake for men and women in just one serving. It is best to choose full-fat, plain yogurt and be sure to check the label to make sure there is no added sugar by way of high-fructose corn syrup or other sweeteners.

Protein Bars

Just like yogurt, some protein bars are formulated to meet low-carb standards, but the majority are not. Many contain as much as 30 grams of sugar per bar, which is equivalent to eating a standard candy bar. If you do enjoy snacking on a protein bar, check the label to ensure that it is high in protein, low in carbohydrates, and low in sugar.

Granola

Granola tends to be classified as a nutritious health food, but most commercial brands include a variety of sweeteners in one package. Cane sugar, brown rice syrup, and tapioca syrup are found in popular commercial selections of granola. Unfortunately, it is commonplace to top flavored yogurt with these sweetened grain mixtures, resulting in a small meal that contains as much as 63 grams of sugar. If you're a granola fan, there are many low-carb renditions that include ingredients such as nuts, seeds, cinnamon, coconut, coconut oil, and vanilla extract, rather than the standard puffed rice, rolled oats, brown sugar, and raisins.

Kombucha

Kombucha is ancient, fermented tea and provides a host of benefits through its probiotic content, however, some brands have as much as 20 grams of sugar per serving, which is almost comparable to the sugar content of soda. If you're looking for the gut and microbiome benefits that kombucha can provide, choose unflavored selections which have less than four grams of sugar per serving.

Cereal Bars

Like cereal, cereal bars are touted as "heart-healthy" yet are packed with added sugars and highly processed ingredients. The nutritional value of the processed ingredients is so low that most cereal bars are fortified with fake synthetic nutrients as the processing kills many of the naturally occurring vitamins and minerals.

Premade Soups

Soups are a wonderful part of the low-carb nutrition plan when using ingredients such as coconut milk, avocado, vegetables, and proteins, however, if you're looking for a quick low-carbohydrate and low-sugar soup found in a can, you will really have to inspect the nutrition label. For example, one can of Campbell's classic tomato soup has 20 grams of sugar—the same as two glazed donuts! Not all canned soups are sugar culprits so with some label checking, you may be able to find some convenient premade options, and remember to choose low-sodium variations if available.

Vitamin Water

Vitamin water is marketed as healthy because it contains a variety of added synthetic nutrients (some of which can be hard to absorb). Another addition to these drinks is sugar—one bottle has as much as 32 grams which is comparable to the amount of sugar found in soda. It's best to stick to water or unsweetened sparkling water on your low-carb nutrition plan.

Canned Baked Beans

Beans and legumes aren't regularly consumed in the low-carb world, however, if you're on point with measuring your carbohydrate intake, you may be able to squeeze a small portion in. This doesn't mean canned baked beans though! Canned baked beans are known for their sweet and tangy flavor because only half a cup packs 10 grams of sugar. Opt for dried beans that you have to prepare yourself so you know there are no added ingredients.

Bottled Smoothies

Many brands of bottled smoothies have more sugar than soda and the misleading factor is their labels are allowed to say, "no added sugars." This is because the sugar technically comes from fruit, however, when several pieces of fruit are processed, stripping their nutrients, and condensed into a bottle, your body cannot decipher this type of sugar from the type found in a candy bar. Smoothies are a part of the low-carb nutrition plan, but opt for ingredients such as coconut milk, kefir, avocado, hemp seeds, kale, and berries.

∗   ∗   ∗

The next contributing factor of our sugar addiction is the fact that there is no guideline or limitation for natural sugar intake—the only limit advised for the public is for added sugars. Referring back to the previous chapter's USDA MyPlate menu, the 108 grams of sugar found in the one-day government-recommended nutrition plan is considered "acceptable" because over 90 percent of those sugars come from "natural" sources, despite the fact that natural sugars are detrimental. The "added sugars" are the only ones tracked and documented by regulatory agencies for the sake of deeming a food acceptable and/or healthy. Since that menu's added sugars do not exceed 10 percent of the daily caloric intake, we will be misled to assume that type of food menu falls within healthy sugar limits, but it certainly does not.

To be clear, added sugars include sugars that are added during the processing of foods, such as white sugar, brown sugar, corn sweetener, corn syrup, dextrose, fructose, glucose, high-fructose corn syrup, lactose, malt syrup, maltose, molasses, raw sugar, and sucrose. While honey and maple syrup are still allowed in many health circles as they're typically considered natural sweeteners, they are so sugar-dense that they are also classified by the FDA as added sugars, as opposed to natural sugars. Most of these added sugars do not include naturally occurring sugars from items such as fruits (fructose) and milk (lactose). What's not being taken into consideration is the fact that the cumulative effect of regular consumption of fructose and lactose, as well as carbohydrates from foods such as breads, cereals, pastas, and potatoes do have adverse effects on blood sugar and make it harder to maintain ideal weight.

In 2016, the FDA amended the requirements for the nutrition label, mandating the listed amounts of added sugars. On one hand, this is a wonderful tool to visualize exactly how much sugar has been added to things like cookies, ice cream, sauces, dressings, and beverages, however, it can also create a false sense of health for a variety of other problematic food choices. If one were faced with a sixteen-ounce orange soda drink which has a label exhibiting 58 grams of added sugar versus a sixteen-ounce orange juice with a label exhibiting 0 added sugars (while still including 48 grams of natural sugar), the "healthy" choice would be the orange juice, as that sugar is "natural." To take this a step further, one may now choose a fruit smoothie that typically has even more sugar than soda, but just as the orange juice, the label will exhibit no added sugars.

Unfortunately, the FDA's "added sugar" label leaves out key information that is detrimental to our health. It does not recognize the fact that the sugars from initial natural fruit sources have been heavily concentrated and processed during production. During this processing, the fruit's properties have been significantly altered, notably the stripping of fiber and concentration of juice from several pieces of fruit into one small bottle. This process greatly affects the way our bodies process the sugar which has key implications for our health, all while leading the consumer to believe he or she is making a healthy choice.[10]

We also come across this same "added sugars" versus "natural sugars" confusion on the nutrition label of dairy products. Lactose, the natural sugar found in milk, has conflicting research regarding how it affects our blood sugar levels. Lactose can, in fact, raise blood glucose levels, however, some nutritionists argue that lactose converts to blood glucose relatively slowly due to the fact that the enzyme lactase slowly splits up glucose into galactose, leading to a slower glycemic response. Other nutrition and medical professionals say that even though dairy has a lower glyemic index ranking, it still stimulates insulin as if it had

10 Marty Micsmeanderings, Evan Lavizadeh, Alireza, Bryan A. Matsumoto, Marco, Emily, et al. "Natural and Added Sugars: Two Sides of the Same Coin," October 5, 2015. http://sitn.hms.harvard.edu/flash/2015/natural-and-added-sugars-two-sides-of-the-same-coin/.

a high glycemic index ranking. This is due to the combination of milk's amino acids found in whey proteins with the lactose. This combination leads some doctors to say that milk's insulin response is actually extreme and should be avoided if one is looking for optimal blood sugar levels.[11]

We have discussed three highly concerning issues that greatly contribute to Americans' collective sugar addiction, as they are very convoluted due to their ambiguous nature. These three findings have a huge impact on the vast majority of the population due to the abundance of use of these hidden-sugar characteristics:

- Manufacturers add sugar to 74 percent of our packaged foods.
- Society labels many sugar-laden foods and nutrition plans as "healthy."
- Natural sugars found in processed foods are viewed as okay as they do not fall in the "added sugar" category, despite having the same health implications as added sugars.

The one and only definitive sugar guideline we are given by the FDA is to limit added sugar intake to 50 grams or less per day, based on a 2,000-calorie diet. Ironically, there is no daily recommended intake for total sugars (added sugars plus natural sugars) because no agency has made the specific recommendation for the amount of total sugars to eat in one day. So essentially, if one consumes 29 grams of added sugars from an eight-ounce soda, 9 grams of added sugar in a serving of breakfast cereal, 8 grams of added sugar in two tablespoons of barbecue sauce, and 4 grams of added sugar in salad dressing, they have remained within the limit of what is deemed a healthy sugar intake by the FDA. Simply adding two sources of natural sugars—milk with the cereal and a fruit smoothie later in the day—brings our total sugars to roughly 120 grams.

---

11 Spero, David. "Is Milk Bad for You? Diabetes and Milk. Diabetes Self Management, June 20, 2017. https://www.diabetes-self-management.com/blog/is-milk-bad-for-you-diabetes-and-milk/.

At the beginning of this chapter, we gave the statistic of 57 pounds of added sugar consumed per year by the average American, but we didn't say how many pounds of total sugars (added plus natural) are consumed on average because that number isn't gauged or monitored since we are not given a guideline for total sugar intake. As nutritionists, we have worked with thousands of clients and have compiled their daily food log questionnaires to try to get a better idea of average total sugar intake— below is an example of a daily meal plan that incorporates the most common meals and snacks.

Standard American Diet Meal Plan

Breakfast
Coffee with flavored creamer
Raisin Bran cereal with milk
Medium banana

Lunch
Turkey sandwich
Chips
Snapple flavored iced tea

Dinner
Chicken with side of pasta and vegetables

Dessert
Serving of ice cream

This common meal plan that, as you can see, seems relatively normal— there's no abundance of sodas, desserts, fried foods, and fast foods—is still not conducive for weight management or health, with 126 grams of sugar (or thirty teaspoons). While some of the sugar content comes from natural sources, this combination of added sugars and natural sugars still results in an overload which is not meant to be tolerated in our bodies. You can assume this sugar number is twofold if one drinks soda regularly

Food	Carbohydrates	Protein	Fat	Sugar
Coffee with flavored creamer (2 tablespoons)	10g	0g	3g	10g
Raisin Bran cereal (1 cup)	46g	5g	2g	18g
2% milk (1 cup)	12g	8g	5g	12g
1 medium banana	23g	1g	0g	12g
Whole wheat bread (2 pieces)	24g	8g	2g	4g
Turkey deli meat (2 pieces)	2g	7g	1g	1g
Cheese (1 piece)	1g	5g	9g	1g
Lettuce, tomato, onion, mustard	6g	0g	0g	2g
Chips (1 small bag)	15g	2g	10g	0g
Snapple peach flavored iced tea (16-ounce bottle)	40g	0g	0g	40g
Chicken (5 ounces)	0g	30g	4g	0g
Broccoli (1 cup)	9g	3g	0g	2g
Whole wheat pasta (1 cup)	41g	7g	2g	2g
Chocolate ice cream (⅔ cup)	23g	3g	11g	22g
Totals	**252g**	**79g**	**49g**	**126g**

and/or indulges in office donuts and cookies, or makes an afternoon run to the local coffee shop for a calorie-ridden pick-me-up.

We want this nutrition plan to help you combat our oversweetened food supply. If you have a sugar addiction, you're not alone. Overcoming the obstacles that have been put in front of us is quite daunting as we can't seem to get away from it—sugar is, in fact, everywhere. If you're finding yourself feeling overwhelmed at the thought of giving up your favorite chocolate or pasta, do not stress, as we have you covered with a *Doctors Weight Loss Diet* shortcut, revealed in the following chapter!

CHAPTER 3
The Low-Carb Solution and the Science Behind It

As previously discussed, sugar is consumed in epic proportions, and that is the number one culprit in weight gain and blood sugar-related ailments. Also, sugar turns to fat if not burned. The second culprit is carbohydrates, as they are sugars that come in two primary forms: simple and complex. Simple carbohydrates include items such as soda, baked goods, packaged cookies, white bread, and some cereals, while complex carbohydrates include foods that have fiber and starch such as potatoes, whole wheat bread, fruits, vegetables, beans, corn, and other grains. The difference between simple and complex carbohydrates is how quickly they digest and absorb, as well as the chemical structure.

When people eat a food containing *any* type of carbohydrate, the digestive system breaks down the digestible ones into sugar, which enters the blood. As blood sugar levels rise, the pancreas produces insulin, a hormone that prompts cells to absorb blood sugar for energy or storage. Mainstream nutrition science advises to consume an average of 275 grams of carbohydrates every day, with the emphasis being on complex carbohydrates. The reasoning behind this is that complex carbohydrates have fiber so they digest more slowly, however, not all complex carbohydrates should be eaten freely while trying to achieve your health and weight loss goals. Just because a particular complex carbohydrate has a bit of fiber, doesn't mean that it will result in a low impact on your blood sugar.

A nutrition tool to use to understand the effects of carbohydrates on your blood sugar is the glycemic index (GI). The glycemic index includes values assigned to foods based on how slowly or how quickly those foods cause increases in blood glucose levels. The ranking system ranges from the numbers 1 to 100 with table sugar being the benchmark for the highest score. Low GI foods have rankings from 1 to 55, medium GI foods have ranking from 56 to 69, and high GI foods have rankings from 70 to 100. According to Harvard Medical School, foods low on the scale tend to release glucose slowly and steadily, and tend to foster weight loss. Foods high on the glycemic index release glucose rapidly.[12] Below you will find the comparison of some common simple and complex carbohydrates, and the GI scores for the "healthy" options may surprise you.

FOOD	Glycemic index (glucose = 100)
High-Carbohydrate Foods	
White bread*	75
Whole wheat bread	74
Unleavened wheat bread	70
Corn tortilla	46
White rice, boiled*	73
Brown rice, boiled	68
Barley	28
Sweet corn	52
Rice noodles†	53
Udon noodles	55
Couscous†	65
Breakfast Cereals	
Cornflakes	81
Wheat flake biscuits	69
Porridge, rolled oats	55
Instant oat porridge	79
Rice porridge/congee	78
Millet porridge	67
Muesli	57

---

12 Harvard Health Publishing, "Glycemic Index for 60+ Foods," Harvard Health, January 6, 2020, https://www.health.harvard.edu/diseases-and-conditions/glycemic-index-and -glycemic-load-for-100-foods.

Fruit and Fruit Products	
Apple, raw†	36
Orange, raw†	43
Avocado	15
Pineapple, raw	59
Mango, raw†	51
Strawberries	41
Grapefruit	25
Blueberries	53
Raspberries	32
Starches	
Potato, boiled	78
Potato, instant mash	87
Potato, French fries	63
Carrots, boiled	39
Sweet potato, boiled	63
Pumpkin, boiled	64
Plantain/green banana	55
Taro, boiled	53
Dairy Products and Alternatives	
Milk, full fat	39
Milk, skim	37
Ice cream	51
Yogurt, fruit	41
Soy milk	34
Rice milk	86
Legumes	
Chickpeas	28
Kidney beans	24
Lentils	32
Green beans	32
Vegetables	
Broccoli	15
Lettuce	15
Cauliflower	10
Asparagus	15

Data are means ± SEM.

* Low-GI varieties were also identified.

† Average of all available data.

For a complete glycemic index, they are easily searchable (and free!) online, but we would like to highlight a few of these carbohydrate comparisons, the first being white bread versus whole wheat bread. We are told by mainstream nutrition science to avoid white bread as it's a simple carbohydrate and will convert to too much sugar, and that whole wheat bread is the better choice. Well, technically, whole wheat (with the GI score of 74) is the "better" choice as the white bread's ranking is 75, but it's still not a healthy choice for weight loss and blood sugar levels as it, too, is high-glycemic. You'll also see the same similarity with white rice (GI score of 73) and brown rice (GI score of 68). Yes, the brown rice is a little bit better than the white rice, but it is on the moderately high end of the scale and will still lead to an ample rise in blood sugar. You'll find another parallel with the cornflakes and wheat flakes cereal—neither are ideal choices, yet wheat cereal is commonly suggested to those who are trying to lose weight or combat type 2 diabetes. All of these carbohydrates are recommended by the governmental nutrition sources since they are supposedly the best choices, while in fact, they are some of the worst.

You may have guessed the solution to this excessive carbohydrate- and sugar-laden lifestyle that many of us have become accustomed to (since it has been recommended for years!) and yes, that is a low-carbohydrate and low-sugar nutrition plan. It is proven nutrition science that low-carbohydrate diets help reduce body weight, heart disease risk factors, bad cholesterol, and blood pressure, and for people with type 2 diabetes, there is reliable evidence that lower carb eating can be safe and useful in lowering average blood glucose levels.[13]

Low-carbohydrate diets have outstanding safety profiles as there have been no reported serious side effects. In fact, many studies demonstrate significant improvements in many important areas. For example, triglycerides (fat in the blood) greatly decrease, while good cholesterol (HDL) increases, and blood pressure and sugar levels greatly decrease as

---

13 Low-Carbohydrate Diets in the Management of Obesity and Type 2 Diabetes: A Review from Clinicians Using the Approach in Practice (nih.gov)

well. Most notably, low-carb diets cause two to three times more weight loss than mainstream low-fat diets that are still being recommended today, and a high percentage of the fat loss comes from the midsection and liver, which substantially lessens the risk for inflammation and disease. Low-carb regimens are particularly effective for those with type 2 diabetes and/or metabolic syndrome.

Low-Carbohydrate Medical Weight Loss Programs

Low-carbohydrate nutrition plans may be intimidating for many since they are so different than what our society is used to eating. After all, eliminating or limiting staples such as bread, cereal, pasta, crackers, rice, and potatoes can seem daunting since we are accustomed to eating these foods throughout the day. You may think there isn't a large enough variety of foods left to choose from if carbohydrate-foods aren't allowed. Chapter 5 will exhibit an array of low-carbohydrate foods you are allotted on the Doctors Weight Loss Diet, and you may be pleasantly surprised! If you're unsure, thinking a diet plan consisting of those foods only may be too difficult to stick to, you may want to consider a medical weight loss

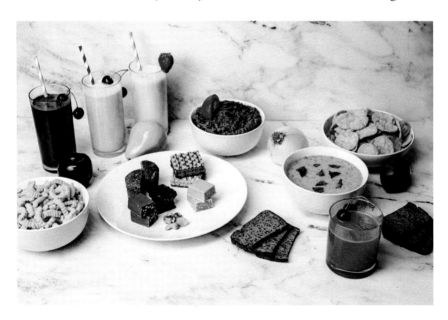

program that boasts packaged foods that only taste like you're cheating. These medical weight loss products consist of items such as bars, shakes, chips, soups, entrées, drinks, and desserts that are formulated to be high in protein, low in carbohydrates, and low in sugar, but still taste like your favorite treats, so it is far easier to adapt to the low-carb lifestyle for many.

It is your decision whether to implement the Doctors Weight Loss Diet via medical-grade weight loss products, or just through typical grocery fare. As you read on, you'll learn how to incorporate the process that is best for your dietary preferences. No matter which route you choose, you are guaranteed to see drastic results if you stick to the plan for as little as thirty days!

CHAPTER 4
Nutrition 101—
Learning the Basics

Welcome to Nutrition 101! Maybe you picked up this book because low-carbohydrate diets yield fast results for millions of people, but if you don't know much about the topic, it may seem daunting to learn. You will be instructed on everything you need to know about nutrition basics so you can apply your knowledge to your eating plan. Weight loss failure is commonly caused by eating the wrong foods that are perceived as healthy, but in fact contribute to weight gain. To fully understand the Doctors Weight Loss protocol, you need to know a little bit about nutrition and dietetics, but not to worry—it's going to be simple and easy to follow. After you get the nutrition basics, the following chapters will tell you everything you can (and can't eat), along with detailed meal plans.

The basic premise of *The Doctors Weight Loss Diet* is to consume foods that are low in carbohydrates and sugar and high in protein. Protein includes amino acids, which are the building blocks of muscle, while sugar and carbohydrates contribute to fat accumulation (if not burned with adequate exercise) so naturally, a diet high in protein and low in sugar and carbohydrates yields results. Of course, we need some carbohydrates, and not all carbs are created equally, but conflicting information in the nutrition world makes it difficult to decipher which carbs will work for us and which will work against us.

Low-Carbohydrate Foods

The Doctors Weight Loss Diet protocol calls for low-carbohydrate, high-protein, and moderate healthy fat intake so the foods you eat will need to reflect this nutrition profile. Generally speaking, you can eat green vegetables, some nongreen vegetables, all animal proteins, some lower-carbohydrate vegan proteins, low-sugar fruits, nuts, seeds, eggs, some dairy, oils, and very limited grains (just for occasional treats). You must limit bread, pasta, potatoes, cereal, crackers, rice, sugar, corn, milk, and other items that are high or moderate in sugar or carbohydrates.

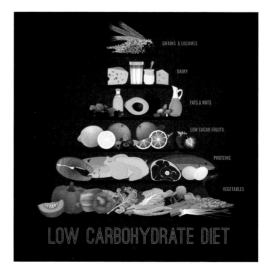

Macronutrients

You will hear this term (or "macros") a lot, and the proper combination of them is the foundation of the diet, so it's important to have a clear understanding of macronutrients. Simply put, macronutrients are fats,

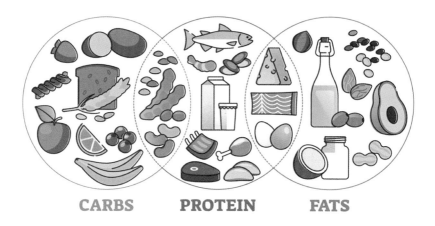

CARBS   PROTEIN   FATS

proteins, and carbohydrates. They are required in large amounts in the diet, hence the term "macro." Macros are measured in grams, such as 40 grams of carbohydrates, 110 grams of protein, and 35 grams of fat. Macronutrients are not to be confused with micronutrients, as micros consist of vitamins and minerals and are needed in the diet in much smaller quantities, so they are measured in the smaller units of milligrams or micrograms.

Low-Carbohydrate Macronutrient Percentages

The Doctors Weight Loss Diet calls for a ratio of macronutrients (fats, proteins, carbohydrates) that have a somewhat flexible range. The percentages require 10 to 20 percent carbohydrates, 50 to 60 percent protein, and 20 to 40 percent fat. This means that most of your calories will come from protein, some will come from healthy fats, and the fewest will come from carbohydrates. The range for carbohydrates provides flexibility, however, the closer you get to 10 percent, the more results you are likely to see. If you are more comfortable in the 20 to 30 percent range for carbs, you will still be consuming around half of what the average American consumes, so you should still expect to achieve your goals.

Calories

As with any nutrition plan, calories in versus calories out will have a bearing on your weight loss and wellness success. It is important to know how many calories you require to hit your personal goals. There are several free online calculators that will reveal how many calories you should consume to get to your goal weight. Once you have determined how many calories you should be consuming, you can refer to the chart on page 27 to see how the Doctors Weight Loss macronutrients align with your caloric intake.

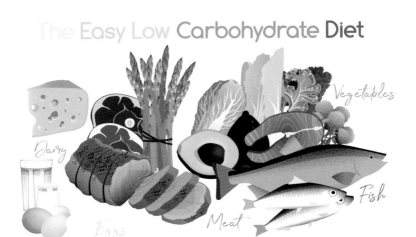

Net Carbohydrates Versus Total Carbohydrates

You will hear talk of "net carbohydrates" in the low-carb nutrition world. Total carbohydrate limits found in the following table account for straight-up carbohydrate totals as listed on the nutrition label. Net carbohydrates are found by subtracting the grams of fiber (which are indigestible carbohydrates) from the grams of carbohydrates. For example, a serving of cauliflower contains five grams of carbohydrates and two grams of fiber so you simply subtract two from five and that gives you three grams of net carbohydrates. Some nutrition circles also advise to subtract grams of sugar alcohols (in addition to the grams of fiber) from the grams of carbohydrates to get net carbohydrates, because sugar alcohols are hard to digest, and therefore are not fully absorbed. If you count total carbohydrates as per the nutrition label, you can follow the table on the next page. If you choose to take the "net carbohydrate" route, an average rule of thumb to follow is to not exceed 25 grams of net carbohydrates per day.

Fats

Many low-carbohydrate diets employ the use of healthy fats, because fat is devoid of sugar. When one eats 50 grams (or less) of carbohydrates per day, they may need to allocate more calories from fat in addition to protein. *The Doctors Weight Loss Diet* calls for low carbohydrates and high

10 to 20 percent carbs, 50 to 60 percent protein, 20 to 40 percent fat

Total Calories	Carbohydrate Calories	Grams of Carbohydrates	Protein Calories	Grams of Protein	Fat Calories	Grams of Fat	Daily Total
1,000	100–200	25–50	500–600	125–150	200–400	22–44	1000 Calories 25–50 grams carbs 125–150 grams protein 22–44 grams fat
1,200	120–240	30–60	600–720	150–180	240–480	27–53	1200 Calories 30–60 grams carbs 150–180 grams protein 27–53 grams fat
1,400	140–280	35–70	700–840	175–210	280–560	31–62	1400 Calories 35–70 grams carbs 175–210 grams protein 31–62 grams fat
1,600	160–320	40–80	800–960	200–240	320–640	36–71	1600 Calories 40–80 grams carbs 200–240 grams protein 36–71 grams protein
1,800	180–360	45–90	900–1080	225–270	360–720	40–80	3000 Calories 233–267 grams fat 75–100 grams protein 38–75 grams carbs

protein, however, how high one chooses to go in protein is a personal choice. Fat will be your lever, as you will increase it if you choose to go lower in protein, and you can decrease it if you prefer higher amounts of protein. Essentially, as long as you stay at 50 grams of carbohydrates (or less), you can alter your fat and protein intake to levels you prefer. Keep in mind, not all fats are created equally, so it is best for your health to limit detrimental fats coming from foods such as bacon, hot dogs, pork rinds, deli meats, and low-carb fast food. Besides the fact that these above-mentioned items can be high in sodium, additives, and preservatives, they also contribute to bad cholesterol and cardiovascular issues. You will want to focus on the healthiest fats which are explained below.

To break it down, omega-6 fatty acids are the most widely consumed in the Western diet as they are found in processed foods by way of soybean oil, corn oil, and safflower oil, as well as cured meats. While we do need to seek these out through foods, since our bodies do not produce them, we eat far too many of them. Omega-3 fatty acids are also essential for the diet since we do not produce them either, but we tend not to get enough omega-3 since they are found in fewer foods. Doctors and dietitians recommend having an omega-6 to omega-3 ratio of no more than 4:1, however, the average ratio in the United States is 50:1, which is a substantial unbalance. When the omega-6 intake far outweighs omega-3, inflammation and inflammatory disease can occur.[14] Adequate omega-3 fatty acid intake is also critical as they are the only fatty acids which contain eicosapentaenoic acid (EPA) and docosahexaenoic acid (DHA). Together, EPA and DHA help to decrease inflammation and heart disease, while on its own, DHA is critical for brain function and eye health. Seafood is the best dietary source of DHA by leaps and bounds and is really the only food which will give adequate amounts of the fatty acid.

Unlike polyunsaturated omega-3 and omega-6, monounsaturated omega-9 fatty acids are actually produced in the body so they are not technically needed in the diet. Research shows that several health

---

14 Calder, P. C.; "Marine Omega-3 Fatty Acids and Inflammatory Processes: Effects, Mechanisms and Clinical Relevance," April 2015, https://pubmed.ncbi.nlm.nih.gov/25149823/.

benefits are associated with replacing inflammatory omega-6 fatty acids with omega-9s. One large-scale study found that higher omega-9 intake reduced plasma triglycerides (fat in the blood) by 19 percent and LDL ("bad") cholesterol by 22 percent in participants with type 2 diabetes.[15] Another study found that people who consumed high-monounsaturated fat diets had better insulin sensitivity, and less inflammation than others who consumed diets high in saturated fat.[16]

For the healthiest and most effective outcomes, consciously opt for more omega-3 and omega-9 fatty acids since they are harder to find in

Foods with Omega-3 Fatty Acids
Salmon
Mackerel
Sardines
Anchovies
Chia seeds
Walnuts
Flax seeds

Foods with Omega-9 Fatty Acids
Olive oil
Cashews and cashew oil
Almonds and almond oil
Avocados and avocado oil
Walnuts and walnut oil

Foods with Omega-6 Fatty Acids
Soybean oil
Corn oil
Standard Mayonnaise
Cottonseed oil
Vegetable oil

---

15 Garg, A.; "High-Monounsaturated-Fat Diets for Patients with Diabetes Mellitus: a Meta-Analysis," March 1998, https://pubmed.ncbi.nlm.nih.gov/9497173/.
16 Finucane, O. M. et al.; "Monounsaturated Fatty Acid-Enriched High-Fat Diets Impede Adipose NLRP3 Inflammasome-Mediated IL-1β Secretion and Insulin Resistance despite Obesity," June 2015, https://pubmed.ncbi.nlm.nih.gov/25626736/.

the diet. You do not need to seek out omega-6 fatty acids as they will naturally fall into place since those are the most common fats in a wide variety of foods. For your convenience, you can refer to the chart on page 29 to see where you can find the different fatty acids.

Proteins

As with fats, it is best to choose the healthiest proteins, so once again, you will want to be conscientiousness about limiting items like processed meats. Opt for unprocessed selections of chicken, turkey, pork, beef, and wild game. In addition, you can find ample protein in other foods such as eggs and dairy products like cheese, cottage cheese, and plain Greek yogurt. Vegan sources of protein include nuts and nut butters, seed and seed butters, cooked spinach, and broccoli. Beans and legumes can be used as a protein source but keep the serving sizes in mind, as you will not want to exceed your daily carbohydrate limit.

Grocery Shopping

It is common misconception that healthier foods which are conducive to weight loss are hard to find, or one must shop at a specialty store. All of your groceries for *The Doctors Weight Loss Diet* can be found at most major grocery stores and many are even quite affordable! You will find an extensive list of all acceptable foods in the following chapter, but generally speaking, your low-carb nutrition plan consists of poultry, seafood, red meat, eggs, cheese, plain yogurt, nuts, nut butters, oils, low-carbohydrate, non-starchy vegetables, and low-sugar fruit.

LOW CARBOHYDRATE DIET
Grocery shopping list

Optimizing your health with:

DAIRY PRODUCTS

SEAFOOD

FISH

MEAT

EGGS

NUTS & SEEDS

FRESH FRUITS & VEGETABLES

LOW CARB

Medical-Grade Weight Loss Product Option

The reason why *The Doctors Weight Loss Diet* is unlike most other low-carbohydrate diets is because you have the option to incorporate already-prepared medical-grade weight loss products. They are formulated to be low in carbohydrates and high in protein while still tasting like your old favorites such as cereal, pasta, cookies, and chocolate. This option is ideal for those who feel they cannot stick solely to a low-carbohydrate diet that incorporates groceries such as the ones listed on the previous page. Research shows that dieters who incorporate medical-grade weight loss products are more likely to maintain the low-carb lifestyle long enough to achieve drastic results simply because, it's just easier! You will find great detail about medical-grade weight loss product meal plans in chapters 7, 8, and 9, and you will find two comparisons of meal plans on the following pages—the first incorporates traditional grocery foods and the second uses medical-grade weight loss products. Following the menus, you will find a breakdown of calories, macronutrients, sodium, fiber, and sugar, so you can see how everything falls into place.

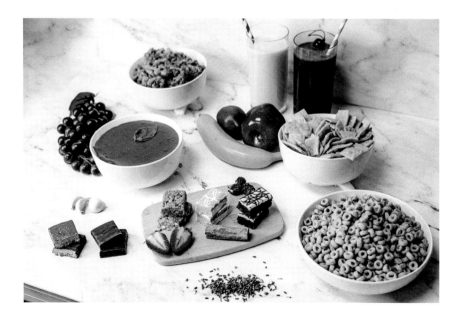

Sample One-Day Meal Plan
(Store-Bought Groceries)

Breakfast: Two whole scrambled eggs and side of raspberries. Coffee with cream or nondairy creamer.

Snack: Serving of almonds.

Lunch: Green salad topped with grilled chicken, diced tomatoes, and onions, and your favorite low-carb, low-sugar salad dressing.

Snack: Celery dipped in hummus.

Dinner: Steak with sautéed mushrooms and broccoli.

Food	Calories	Fat	Protein	Net Carbs	Sodium	Fiber	Sugar
Eggs (2 whole)	156	10g	12g	1g	124mg	0g	0g
Raspberries (½ cup)	33	0g	0g	3g	0mg	4g	3g
Cream (1 tablespoon)	20	2g	0g	0g	5mg	0g	0g
Almonds (23 whole)	164	14g	6g	3g	0mg	4g	0g
Romaine lettuce (2 cups)	16	0g	1g	1g	8mg	2g	1g
Chicken breast (1 cup, chopped)	231	5g	38g	0g	104mg	0g	0g
Diced tomatoes (¼ cup)	8	0g	0g	1g	2mg	0.5g	1g
Diced onions (2 tablespoons)	8	0g	0g	2g	1mg	0g	1g
Low-carb salad dressing (2 tablespoons)	50	5g	0g	2g	140mg	0g	0g
Celery (2 stalks)	11	0g	1g	1g	64mg	1g	0g
Hummus (2 tablespoons)	50	3g	2g	2g	57mg	2g	0g
Sirloin Steak (8 ounces)	414	13g	65g	0g	72mg	0g	0g
Sautéed mushrooms (½ cup)	38	2g	1g	3g	25mg	0g	0g
Broccoli (1 cup)	62	0g	3g	7g	60mg	5g	2g
Totals	**1,261**	**54g**	**129g**	**26g**	**662mg**	**18.5g**	**8g**

Sample One-Day Meal Plan
(Medical-Grade Weight Loss Products)

Breakfast: Medical-grade high-protein, low-carbohydrate blueberry pancakes.

Snack: Medical-grade high-protein, low-carbohydrate pretzel twists dipped in mashed avocado.

Lunch: Medical-grade high-protein, low-carbohydrate cheesesteak pasta.

Snack: Medical-grade high-protein, low-carbohydrate vanilla wafers.

Dinner: Grilled chicken with a side roasted cauliflower topped with shredded cheese, and a side salad with low-carb dressing.

Food	Calories	Fat	Protein	Net Carbs	Sodium	Fiber	Sugar
High-protein pancakes (1 serving)	90	0.5g	15g	6g	260mg	1g	1g
High-protein pretzels (1 serving)	120	3g	12g	7g	320mg	4g	1g
Mashed avocado (4 tablespoons)	110	10g	2g	0g	0mg	6g	0g
High-protein pasta (1 serving)	140	2.5g	12g	13g	480mg	3g	2g
High-protein vanilla wafers (1 serving)	200	9g	15g	13g	75mg	0g	6g
Grilled chicken (6 ounces)	276	6g	52g	0g	90mg	0g	0g
Cauliflower (1 cup florets)	29	0.5g	2g	2g	19mg	3g	3g
Cheddar cheese (¼ cup, grated)	114	9g	6g	1g	184mg	0g	0g
Romaine lettuce (2 cups, chopped)	16	0g	0.5g	0.5g	4mg	1g	0.5g
Low-carb salad dressing (2 tablespoons)	50	5g	0g	2g	140mg	0g	0g
Totals	**1145**	**45.5g**	**116.5g**	**44.5g**	**1572mg**	**18g**	**13.5g**

As you can see from the two sample meals plans, both are very low in carbohydrates and sugar, which will lead to dramatic weight loss results. The primary difference is by integrating medical-grade weight loss products, you do not have to give up foods such as pancakes, pretzels, pasta, and treats as they are specially formulated to be low in carbohydrates and sugar. You will learn more about these products (and if they are right for you) in chapter 6's preparation phase questionnaire.

We hope this chapter has given you the basic understanding and foundation of the low-carb protocol. Simply put, make sure you're consuming 10 to 20 percent carbohydrates, 50 to 60 percent protein, and 20 to 40 percent healthy fats. This regimen will put you on the fast track to weight loss and stabilized blood sugar levels, but remember it's not required to track to your calories and macronutrients—but if you prefer to, contact us at info@doctorsweightloss.com for your complimentary nutrition tracker application. To see exactly what you can (and can't) eat, read on to the next chapter!

CHAPTER 5

Everything You Can (and Can't) Eat

This chapter is your go-to guide for everything you can and can't eat to achieve your low-carbohydrate nutrition plan. The meal plans found in coming chapters do not include every single item in the following "can" list, however, more options are listed in case you are looking for a variety of additions. The following lists contain the lowest-carbohydrate foods in each category so these selections should be the foundation of your nutrition protocol.

A NOTE ABOUT ORGANIC PRODUCE

It is always best to purchase as much organic produce as possible to avoid toxins and pesticides, but it can get pricey! There is a small handful of low-carbohydrate vegetables and fruits that fall into the "dirty dozen" category, meaning they have the highest levels of pesticides. If possible, it is best to purchase the organic variations of these "dirty dozen" selections and we have highlighted those for you.

A NOTE ABOUT ONIONS

A 100-gram (⅔ cup) serving of onions/shallots can have as much as 17 grams of carbohydrates, however, the manner in which one typically eats onions calls for much less than that. When sprinkling onions on a salad or sautéing shallots for a sauce, the carbohydrate count is still low enough. If you're eating a roasted vegetable mixture and one component is onion, try not to exceed more than ½ cup of the onions.

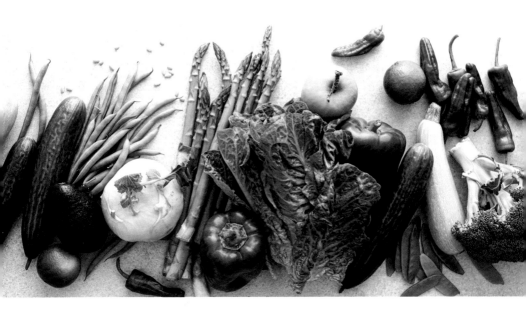

Vegetables

If you're unsure of which vegetables are best when making a grocery run, sticking to selections that are green is a rule to keep in mind. If you don't see your favorite(s) on the list, you can add them to the "can" category if green in color. If they are not green, check to see if each serving has 5 grams or less of net carbohydrates.

Artichokes	Fennel bulb
Arugula	Green beans
Asparagus	Hot peppers
Bok Choy	Kale
Broccoli	Kohlrabi
Broccoli Rabe	Lettuces
Brussels sprouts	Mushrooms
Cabbage/sauerkraut	Onions
Cauliflower	Radishes
Celery	Seaweed
Chard	Spinach
Chicory greens	Swiss chard
Endive	Watercress

The Doctors Weight Loss Diet

Fruits

Some low-sugar fruits are allowed for regular consumption as they are extremely low in carbohydrates, and some are so low in sugar that we may think of them as vegetables as opposed to fruits. Many fruits such as mango and grapes contain high amounts of fructose, which affects our bodies in a similar manner as table sugar so it is imperative to eliminate high-glycemic fruits while adhering to your low-carb plan. Below are approved fruits for you to incorporate on a regular basis.

Avocados	Olives
Bell peppers (any color)	Pumpkin
Blackberries	Raspberries
Blueberries	Spaghetti squash
Cucumbers/pickles	Strawberries
Eggplant	Tomatoes
Lemons	Zucchini
Limes	

A NOTE ABOUT BERRIES

Berries are relatively low in sugar and carbohydrates, compared to many other varieties of fruit, and they are packed with essential micronutrients, fiber, and antioxidants, so they are a healthy addition to anyone's diet. Since we are trying to remain extremely low in sugar and carbohydrates, this table will help you to be mindful of your berry intake.

50-gram (½ cup) serving		
Berry Type	**Total Carbs**	**Net Carbs**
Blackberries	5g	2.5g
Raspberries	6g	2.5g
Strawberries	4g	3g
Blueberries	10.5g	8.5g

COOKING OILS AND FATS

Type	Smoke Point	Uses	Health Benefits
Olive oil	325–405°F	Low and medium heat cooking, "finishing oil" for flavor, salad dressings, marinades, drizzling over lettuces and vegetables.	High in monounsaturated fats which is linked to lower blood pressure and cholesterol. Consumption linked with improved cognitive health and blood vessel function, and the manufacturing process does not employ chemicals.
Coconut oil	350°F	Roasting at low temperatures, baking, smoothie, shake, or coffee addition; can be substituted in for butter and other oils with a 1:1 ratio.	Provides easily absorbed medium chain fatty acids (MCTs) which are conducive for ketosis. Anti-inflammatory properties and beneficial for gut health.
Medium Chain Triglyceride (MCT) oil	320°F	Used as a supplement and not typically for cooking; ingredient in salad dressings, smoothies, shakes, and keto coffee.	Higher amount of MCTs than coconut oil—these saturated fats are easily digested and conducive for achieving ketosis. Beneficial for energy, and the feeling of satiety.
Avocado oil	520°F	Ideal for grilling, roasting, and panfrying due to high smoke point. Can also be drizzled on salads and vegetables, or as a mayonnaise replacement to add creaminess to dressings, sauces, and dips.	Monounsaturated fat to promote good cholesterol and heart health. Provides vitamin E, antioxidants, and healthy fats.
Walnut oil	320°F	Not ideal for cooking due to low smoke point. Can be added to shakes, smoothies, dressing, sauces, and keto coffee.	Good source of omega-3 fats which is beneficial for heart, eye, and brain health. The fats found in walnut oil can help reduce bad cholesterol and increase good cholesterol.

The Doctors Weight Loss Diet

COOKING OILS AND FATS			
Type	Smoke Point	Uses	Health Benefits
Grass-fed butter	300 to 350°F	Used for low-heat cooking of eggs, fish, or shellfish. Topper for steak, roasted veggies, or keto chaffles.	Grass-fed butter has a higher composition of omega-3 fatty acids compared to grain-fed butter. Omega-3s are beneficial for heart and brain health, and cholesterol.
Grass-fed ghee	485°F	Used for sautéing meat, poultry, seafood, and vegetables. Can replace butter in most recipes, or be used as a spread.	Ghee is clarified butter so it is lactose- and casein-free, while still having a buttery taste and texture.

Proteins

You will find a variety of animal proteins in this section but some selections have more fat content than others, so keep in mind that more fat means more calories since one gram of protein has four calories, and one gram of fat has nine calories. We are mainly concerned about carbohydrates since carbs turn into sugar, so don't feel as if you need to steer clear from the fattier selections. All animal proteins that have a substantial fat content are marked as such for your convenience.

Poultry	Eggs	Red Meat
Chicken	Chicken eggs	Beef
Chicken with skin	Duck eggs	Boar
Duck	Goose eggs	Buffalo
Game hen	Quail eggs	Elk
Pheasant		Goat
Quail		Lamb
Rabbit		Pork/Bacon/Sausage
Turkey		Venison
Turkey with skin		

Seafood

Anchovies	Halibut	Sardines
Bass	Herring	Scallops
Carp	Lobster	Snails
Catfish	Mackerel	Snapper
Clams	Mussels	Sole
Cod	Octopus	Swordfish
Crab	Oysters	Trout
Flounder	Prawns	Tuna
Haddock	Salmon	Walleye

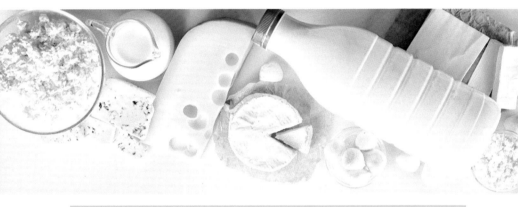

Dairy

Butter and Ghee (clarified butter)	Feta	Greek yogurt (full-fat)
Cheeses	Goat cheese	Half-and-half
Blue cheese	Gouda	Heavy whipping cream
Brie	Gruyère	
Camembert	Mascarpone	Kefir
Cheddar	Mozzarella	Sour cream (full-fat)
Cottage cheese (full-fat)	Muenster	
Cream cheese (full-fat)	Parmesan	
	Provolone	
	Ricotta	
	Swiss	

Nuts, Seeds, Nut Butters, Seed Butters

Some nuts and seeds are lower in carbohydrates and higher in fat, making them better choices, however, all selections below are allowed on your low-carb nutrition plan. The lowest-carbohydrate selections are Brazil nuts, macadamia nuts, and pecans, while the highest in carbohydrates are cashews and pistachios. All others fall somewhere in between.

Almonds	Pine nuts	Almond butter
Brazil nuts	Pistachios	Cashew butter
Cashews	Walnuts	Hemp seed butter
Coconut	Chia seeds	Macadamia butter
(unsweetened)	Flax seeds	Peanut butter
Hazelnuts	Hemp seeds	Pecan butter
Macadamia nuts	Poppy seeds	Sesame seed butter
Peanuts	Pumpkin seeds	Walnut butter
Pecans	Sesame seeds	
Pili nuts	Sunflower seeds	

Dressings and Sauces

There are many dressings and sauces that are allowed on the low-carb nutrition plan, so there is no need to worry about a shortage of flavor. The following premade selections can be found in most grocery stores but make sure to check the ingredients labels to ensure they have no (or very little) sugar. If you prefer to make your own dressings and sauces, please refer to chapter 24.

Aioli	Hot sauce	Mustard
Alfredo	Italian dressing	Pesto
Bearnaise	Ketchup (sugar-free	Ranch dressing
Blue cheese dressing	only)	Soy sauce
Buffalo sauce	Marinara sauce (no	Sriracha
Caesar dressing	added sugars)	Tzatziki
Gorgonzola sauce	Mayonnaise (avocado	
Hollandaise	oil and regular)	

Miscellaneous Pantry Items

Anchovy paste
Apple cider vinegar
Balsamic vinegar
Bouillon cubes
Broth
Capers
Chocolate (at least
    75 percent cacao)
Coconut cream
Coconut milk (full
    fat)
Curry paste
Fish sauce
Red wine vinegar
Tomato paste (low-
    carb, sugar-free)
Vanilla extract

Beverages

Water
Sparkling water
Flavored sparkling water
    (sugar-free)
Fruit-infused water (pitcher
    of water with lemon, lime,
    cucumber, etc.)
Unsweetened coffee
Keto coffee
Unsweetened tea
Kombucha (low-sugar only)

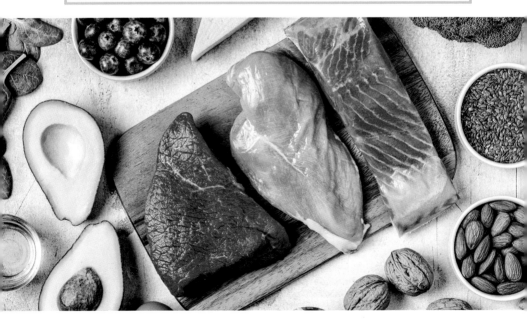

The Doctors Weight Loss Diet

Wine and Liquor

You can still participate in happy hour or have an adult beverage after a long day of work while on your low-carb plan. While some alcoholic drinks are packed with sugar and carbohydrates, others have the proper macros to fit into your nutrition plan if consumed in moderation. Having one (or sometimes two) of the following low-sugar and low-carbohydrate beverages occasionally won't sabotage your goals.

Red Wine	White Wine	Liquor
Cabernet Sauvignon	Albarino	Brandy
Merlot	Brut Champagne	Gin
Petite Syrah	Chardonnay	Rum
Pinot Noir	Pinot Blanc	Tequila
Syrah	Pinot Grigio	Vodka
Zinfandel	Sauvignon Blanc	Whisky

You may be pleasantly surprised that such a large variety of foods is allowed on the low-carb nutrition plan. And of course, you are not required to use all of these foods, but they are available if you should choose to add them to your grocery cart. Now you will find the foods to limit and eliminate. The two common denominators which put foods on the limitation/exclusion lists are sugar and carbohydrate contents that are too high for the low-carb protocol. Given that on average you'll be staying under 50 grams of total carbohydrates per day, **you can potentially consume some of the foods in the orange list on page 44, in moderation** (no more than three servings per week) as they have between 8 and 20 grams of carbohydrates per serving. **The red listed foods to eliminate should be avoided** most of the time since they are the highest in carbohydrates and sugar, but of course, if you're having a special occasion like a birthday, have a piece of cake and jump right back on the wagon!

Occasional Foods

The following foods are a hot topic in the low-carb world. On one hand, they boast excellent nutritional properties that are beneficial to have in anyone's diet plan. On the other hand, their carbohydrate content is considered to be too high in many circles. You can still fit an occasional serving in (no more than three times per week) and remain within your macronutrient goals, so while you shouldn't consume these foods on a regular basis, you can have a portioned serving periodically.

Sweet potato   Lentils
Quinoa   Oatmeal
Beans   Butternut squash
Peas   All fruits

Foods to Eliminate

White and whole   Pizza crust   Corn
  wheat bread Croissants   Cow's milk
White and whole   Muffins   Soda
  wheat pasta Pita bread   Fruit juice and other
Cereal   Pita chips   sugary beverages
Crackers   Potato chips   Candy
Rice   White and whole   Cookies
Tortilla   wheat flour Cake
Commercial granola   Bagels   Donuts
  bars   White potatoes   Ice cream

---

*   The best low-carb mixers are club soda, plain sparkling water, and lime juice.

CHAPTER 6
The Preparation Phase (Don't Skip this Chapter!)

First of all, congratulations for taking the first step in your health and weight loss journey! This chapter will not only prepare you for your nutrition regimen but it will also assist you with choosing the proper protocol based on your individualized needs and goals. In very general terms, you will find two entirely different ways to adopt your new low-carbohydrate, high-protein lifestyle. One being through use of medical-grade weight loss products, and the other being through typical fare you find at the grocery store. In order to determine which route may be best for you, see the dieter profile types below and choose the one which resonates with you.

Dieter Profile A
- Wants a straightforward, easy-to-follow plan.
- Wants to be told exactly what to eat to achieve results.
- Needs structure.
- Does not enjoy cooking or does not have time to cook.
- Has a very busy schedule.
- Needs help with accountability.
- Enjoys packaged foods that can be taken on the go.
- Is likely to fall off the wagon without sweet and/or savory treats.
- Is uncertain about which foods will assist with weight loss.
- Does not want to be forced to exercise to achieve results.

Dieter Profile B

- Does not mind grocery shopping, food prepping, and cooking.
- Has some time to spend in the kitchen.
- Ability to achieve results without a lot of structure.
- Has personal accountability.
- Does not consume packaged foods.
- Prefers to eat typical fare from grocery stores.
- Does not mind packing healthy snacks to take on the go.
- Does not want to be forced to exercise to achieve results.

If Dieter Profile A is more closely matched to your own opinions and needs, a structured medical-grade weight loss program may help you achieve your results the most quickly and efficiently. If Dieter Profile B is a closer match to your lifestyle and preferences, a low-carbohydrate, high-protein regimen, consisting of standard grocery fare meal plans may be more suited for you. Preparation Phase Part One (directly below) will be for both Dieters A and B, and then Preparation Phase Part Two will branch off, listing completely different prep phase tasks for each dieter.

Preparation Phase Part One (for both Dieters A and B)

Clean Out Your Kitchen

We know this can be difficult but your chances of success skyrocket if there are no temptations nearby. We don't necessarily suggest being wasteful, but taking a stand and dumping cookies, chips, and soda into the garbage is a surefire way to kick off your new lifestyle in a determined fashion. Or you can give your treats away to family and friends while declaring your new lifestyle and you may be surprised to find that instead of taking you up on your generous offerings, a friend or two may find inspiration and join you on the journey. If suddenly clearing the decks is feeling a little too abrupt and nerve-racking, simply have a last hurrah and start your new meal plan after all of the treats are gone (but don't buy anymore at the store, in the meantime)! For your low-carbohydrate lifestyle, you'll want to dispose of, give away, or finish off and not rebuy the following items:

FOODS TO ELIMINATE

White and whole
  wheat bread
White and whole
  wheat pasta
Cereal
Crackers
Rice
Tortilla
Commercial granola
  bars

Pizza crust
Croissants
Muffins
Pita bread
Pita chips
Potato chips
White and whole
  wheat flour
Bagels
White potatoes

Corn
Cow's milk
Soda
Fruit juice and other
  sugary beverages
Candy
Cookies
Cake
Donuts
Ice cream

You May Want to Weigh In!

If you don't have a scale, it is beneficial to purchase one so you can track your progress, and it doesn't need to be anything fancy or expensive—just a simple scale that measures your weight. If you have access to a gym scale and you use the gym somewhat regularly, that can work too. Weight fluctuates throughout the day due to water and food consumption, as well as the clothing we're wearing, so we recommend weighing in first thing in the morning before getting dressed for the day. Jot your weight down or put it in your phone. When you complete your second weigh-in, consistency is key, so if on your first weigh-in, you stepped on the scale before eating anything and before getting dressed in the morning, do the same for all further weigh-ins, making them all consistent by following those guidelines.

Before Pictures

Sometimes we get just as much (or even more) results from inches lost, as opposed to the number on the scale. In addition to weighing in, take three before pictures—one frontward facing, one side facing, and one from behind. At the end of each thirty days, you can take the same three pictures so you can visually see the progress you have made. If you want to share your success, tag @dwlteam on Instagram and @DoctorsWeightLossFB on Facebook, so everyone can see your results!

Tracking System Application (for both Dieters A and B)

You may have heard of (or even used) calorie and macronutrient tracking systems such as MyFitnessPal, FatSecret, and Carb Manager, but Doctors Weight Loss has its own and since you have purchased this book, you can contact us at info@doctorsweightloss.com for complimentary access to the application. Our system includes a database of the Doctors Weight Loss medical-grade weight loss products as well as over 6,000 grocery foods so no matter which plan you choose, the tracker will be perfect for you. In addition to tracking calories and macros, this comprehensive application can be accessed by your smartphone or desktop computer, allowing you to gauge your water intake, exercise, sleep, and more!

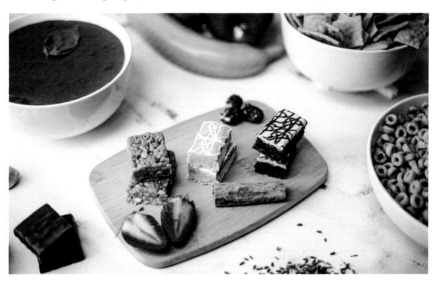

Dieter A Preparation Phase Part Two

Based on your own profile being closer to Dieter A's needs and preferences, a medical-grade weight loss program that includes the use of formulated packaged products may be the most beneficial for achieving your goals. If after reading through this chapter, you determine that the plan for Dieter B may be up your alley, by all means, feel free to go that route. This accelerated plan for Dieter A is extremely straightforward and structured and lays out exactly what to eat everyday; average success is a fifteen-pound loss in one month. Your typical day of food will look like this:

Accelerated Plan Allowance per Day

3–4 medical-grade weight loss products
2–3 servings low-carbohydrate vegetables
1 serving low-sugar fruit (optional)
1 serving healthy fat (optional)
6–8 ounces quality protein

You may be wondering what the previously mentioned medical-grade weight loss products are, exactly. These products are prepackaged foods such as shakes, bars, cereals, pancakes, chips, snacks, entrées, pastas, soups, drinks, and desserts. They are specially formulated for weight loss, averaging 150 calories, 15 grams of protein, and 4 grams of carbohydrates per serving. The three primary brands we recommend are Nutriwise, Protiwise, and BestMed, which are used in hospitals and weight loss clinics around the world and are implemented by physicians as their protocol for patients. The three different

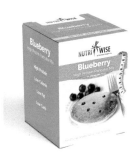

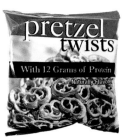

brands are formulated very similarly with only some variation in ingredients, fiber, vitamins, and minerals, and the hundreds of products found among the three brands provide variety for use throughout the day from breakfast to an after-dinner dessert. In this chapter you will find example combinations of products from each line but keep in mind, you can mix and match!

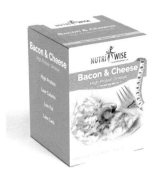

In addition to your four medical-grade weight loss products, you will also consume two to three servings of low-carbohydrate vegetables, six to eight ounces of quality protein, one optional healthy fat, and one optional serving of low-sugar fruit per day. Those additional foods can be consumed in a variety of different ways, and at different times of the day, in conjunction with your weight loss products. The following chapter will outline a detailed accelerated meal plan, so feel free to skip ahead before you decide which products you will incorporate into your daily regimen.

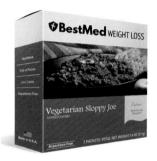

How to Order Your Products

You will find the Nutriwise, Protiwise, and BestMed medical-grade weight loss products online at doctorsweightloss .com and they will be shipped directly to you. You can choose all products from

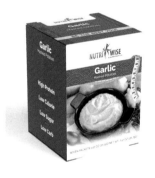

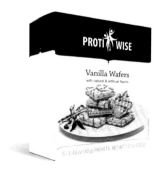

one of the above-mentioned brands or you can mix and match, as they are all formulated to be low in carbohydrates and sugar and high in protein. Hundreds of thousands of dieters have used these products to lose an average of fifteen pounds per month, but as much as twenty-five pounds per month for many. The number of products you will need depends on the plan you choose. The following chapters detail the Accelerated, Lifestyle, and Maintenance plans, and list how many products are needed and how to incorporate them into your specific meal plan.

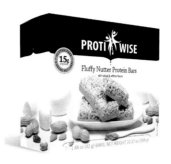

Dieter B Preparation Phase Part Two

Based on your own profile being closer to Dieter B's needs and preferences, your low-carb nutrition plan will not contain any medical-grade weight loss products—it will only consist of standard grocery fare. Keep in mind, if you're looking for an easy on-the-go high-protein, low-carb snack, you can certainly integrate a medical-grade weight loss product (or two) into your daily plan. Refer to the maintenance plan in chapter 9 to learn how!

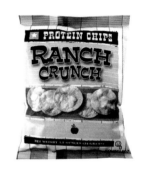

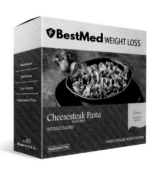

If after reading through this chapter, you determine that the plan for Dieter A may be up your alley, by all means, feel free to go that route. After completing the initial preparation tasks found in this chapter

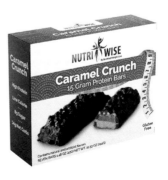

(cleaning out your kitchen, weighing in, and taking before pictures), you will dive right into grocery shopping and meal planning. So you're not wasting any time reading this whole book if you'd prefer to skip ahead and jump right into your new low-carb life via typical foods you can find in most mainstream grocery stores to fast-track your way to your new body, just focus on the following chapters:

Chapter 5: Everything You Can (and Can't) Eat
Chapter 10: The Fastest and Easiest Way to Start Your New Low-Carb Life
Chapter 11: The Low-Carb Seven-Day Meal Plan Photo Guide
Chapter 12: Low-Carb Food Groups and Servings
Chapter 13: The Low-Carb Select Meal Planning System

We hope this chapter has helped you decide how to proceed with your weight loss plan—an approach that incorporates low-carb, high-protein medical-grade weight loss products, or one that derives a low-carb, high-protein regimen only from standard grocery fare. The primary reasons dieters choose plans that incorporate products is because of convenience and the ability to still eat favorite foods such as pasta, cereal, chips, and desserts—it makes the transition into the low-carb lifestyle that much easier. If you prefer standard low-carb grocery foods such as vegetables, proteins, healthy fats, and low-sugar fruits, and don't mind spending a little more time in the kitchen, reference the above listed chapters first!

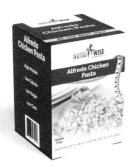 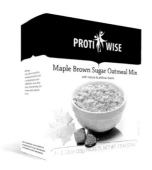 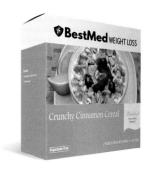

IMPORTANT NOTE

No matter which plan you choose (Accelerated, Lifestyle, or Maintenance), make sure you get acquainted with this quick guide to acceptable foods!

Below you will find a snapshot of choices of foods for the vegetable, low-sugar fruit, and protein categories, however, all options listed in chapter 5 are acceptable. If you're unsure about portions, feel free to use the following table as a general guide, however, if you need a little more protein or vegetables, you may go beyond these limits by a few ounces, or by ½ to 1 full cup. Please adhere to the low-sugar fruit serving maximum for the best results.

Vegetables: 1 cup
Leafy Greens: 2 cups
Low-Sugar Fruits: ½ cup
Quality Protein: 6–8 ounces
Healthy Fats: Vary by type (see below)

Vegetables/Leafy Greens: Kale, broccoli, spinach, collard greens, lettuce, asparagus, artichoke, Brussels sprouts, raw carrots, celery, or any green vegetable. There is no need to be overly particular about what types of vegetables you consume as long as you do not include corn or potatoes.

Low-Sugar Fruits: Blueberries, raspberries, blackberries, strawberries, onions, bell peppers, eggplant, tomato, olives, avocado.

Quality Proteins: Whole eggs, chicken, turkey, fish, shellfish, lean beef, quinoa, beans, peas, lentils, nuts, seeds, cottage cheese, Greek yogurt, broccoli, cooked spinach. If you are choosing beans, peas, lentils, or quinoa, no more than four ounces per day due to carbohydrate content.

Healthy Fats: Avocado (½ of a whole), healthy oils (1 tablespoon), coconut, olives (5–7 whole), salmon (6–8 ounces), eggs (1–2 whole), nuts and seeds (¼ cup), nut and seed butters (2 tablespoons), whole fat Greek yogurt (½ cup), cheese in moderation (1.5 ounces).

Drinks: Water, coffee, or tea with cream or nondairy creamer, but no sugar added. Fruit-infused water (place a pitcher of water with favorite sliced fruits in the refrigerator and let sit for a few hours)—some examples are cucumber/orange/mint, lemon by itself, grapefruit by itself, and orange by itself. Carbonated drinks such as La Croix or sparkling water with a bit of flavor are permitted.

Use Your Oils Every Day!

Aside from the one optional serving of healthy fat, the oils found in chapter 5 should be used regularly for cooking and dressing purposes, as these types of fats assist with blood sugar regulation, craving prevention, and good cholesterol. Oils can be used for roasting, sautéing, vegetable topping, and salad dressing (you can combine with vinegar). If you prefer store-bought dressing, be sure to check the nutrition label and choose ones that have no more than 3 grams of sugar and/or 3 grams of carbohydrates per two-tablespoon serving.

CHAPTER 7

Doctors Weight Loss Accelerated Plan

If you have chosen to take the accelerated route to jump-start your weight loss, this chapter will outline exactly what to eat. First of all, you need 120 units of medical-grade weight loss products that will allow four pre-packaged products per day, along with one sensible meal consisting of vegetables, proteins, and an optional low-sugar fruit. When ordering your products at doctorsweightloss.com, keep in mind that most boxes contain seven units of products, however, a handful contain only five units. If you're ordering all boxes with seven units, you'll need (roughly) seventeen boxes of products, but remember to adjust accordingly if you order a five-unit box.

The Accelerated Plan is exactly how it sounds—it produces the fastest results! Feel free to adhere to this plan until you get to your goal weight and then use the following chapters to wean off gradually and establish your grocery-based low-carbohydrate lifestyle. Not only is the Accelerated Plan highly effective, it's also extremely simple, as you are allowed the adjacent list of foods each day. The two to three servings of vegetables, one optional low-sugar fruit, and six to eight ounces of protein can be eaten all in one meal, or spread out through the day however you desire.

Accelerated Plan Allowance per Day

3–4 Medical-grade weight loss products
2–3 servings low-carbohydrate vegetables
1 serving low-sugar fruit (optional)
1 serving healthy fat (optional)
6–8 ounces quality protein

Below you will find **three sample visual meal plans** that follow the above-mentioned guidelines. The first four photos are of the actual Doctors Weight Loss (DWL) medical-grade products, and you will see they look (and taste) just like your old favorites. The last photo is of the sensible meal you will be responsible for preparing—that meal incorporates the protein, vegetables, and optional heathy fat and fruit. Further into this chapter, you will find a sample 21-day accelerated meal plan.

Sample Accelerated Meal Plan One

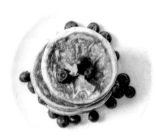

DWL high-protein pancakes

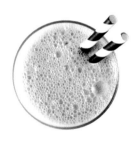

DWL high-protein
strawberry shake

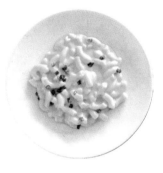

DWL high-protein pasta

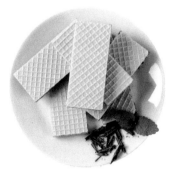

DWL vanilla wafers

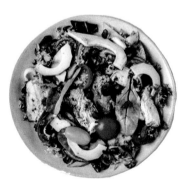

Sensible meal

Sample Accelerated Meal Plan Two

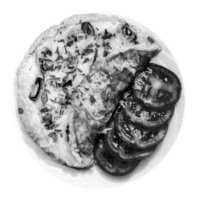

DWL high-protein omelet

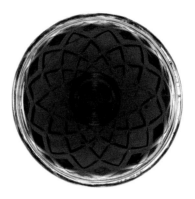

DWL high-protein jello

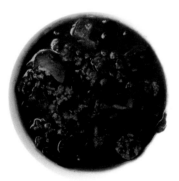

DWL high-protein chili

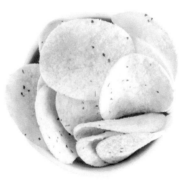

DWL high-protein chips

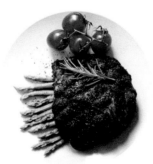

Sensible meal

Sample Accelerated Meal Plan Three

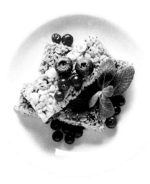

DWL high-protein bar

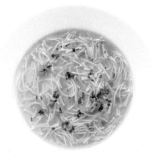

DWL high-protein soup

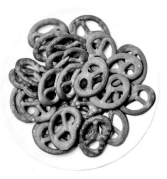

DWL high-protein snack

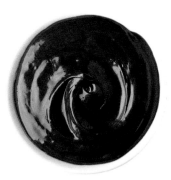

DWL high-protein pudding

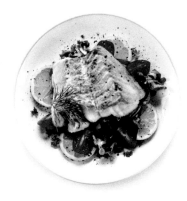

Sensible meal

Now let's put all of these guidelines in place to exhibit a typical 21-day accelerated plan. If you have a busy schedule and only want to focus on products throughout the day and leave the food preparation to dinner only, you will find those examples from Days 1 through 8. You will see that Days 8 through 14 incorporate different combinations of the fruit, vegetable, and fat options throughout the day. Keep in mind, you are not required to choose dinner as your one meal to prepare—if you prefer to make breakfast or lunch as your main meal of the day instead, you will find those options in Days 15 through 21. Simply choose your favorite method and stick to it!

DAY 1	DAY 2
Breakfast: DWL product	**Breakfast:** DWL product
Snack: DWL product	**Snack:** DWL product
Lunch: DWL product	**Lunch:** DWL product
Snack: DWL product	**Snack:** DWL product
Dinner: Grilled/roasted chicken (protein) with green beans (low-carb vegetable), side salad (low-carb vegetable), topped with half an avocado (healthy fat)	**Dinner:** Bun-less burger (protein) topped with cheese (fat), lettuce/tomato/onion (vegetable and fruit), with a side of roasted broccoli (low-sugar ketchup, mustard, and mayonnaise are optional)
DAY 3	DAY 4
Breakfast: DWL product	**Breakfast:** DWL product
Snack: DWL product	**Snack:** DWL product
Lunch: DWL product	**Lunch:** DWL product
Snack: DWL product	**Snack:** DWL product
Dinner: Grilled fish of choice (protein) with grilled asparagus (vegetable), served with avocado oil mayonnaise to dip (fat), with side salad (vegetable)	**Dinner:** Steak (protein) topped with sautéed mushrooms (low-carb produce), and a side of sautéed spinach (vegetable)

DAY 5	DAY 6
Breakfast: DWL product	**Breakfast:** DWL product
Snack: DWL product	**Snack:** DWL product
Lunch: DWL product	**Lunch:** DWL product
Snack: DWL product	**Snack:** DWL product
Dinner: Roasted turkey (protein) with green beans (vegetable) and mashed cauliflower (vegetable), topped with shredded cheese (fat)	**Dinner:** Pork chops (protein) with sauerkraut (vegetable) and side salad (vegetable), topped with avocado (fat)
DAY 7	**DAY 8**
Breakfast: DWL product	**Breakfast:** DWL product
Snack: DWL product	**Snack:** ½ cup blueberries (low-sugar fruit)
Lunch: DWL product	**Lunch:** DWL product with a side salad (low-sugar vegetable)
Snack: DWL product	**Snack:** DWL product and handful of almonds (healthy fat)
Dinner: Sautéed shrimp (protein) with a side of riced cauliflower (vegetable), topped with shredded cheddar or grated Parmesan cheese (fat), and a side of sautéed bok choy (vegetable)	**Dinner:** Grilled chicken breast (quality protein) with Brussels sprouts (low-sugar vegetable)
	Dessert: DWL product
DAY 9	**DAY 10**
Breakfast: DWL product	**Breakfast:** DWL product
Snack: Raw carrot sticks (low-sugar vegetable) dipped in mashed avocado (healthy fat)	**Snack:** Celery sticks (low-sugar vegetable) dipped in real peanut or almond butter (healthy fat)
Lunch: DWL product	**Lunch:** DWL product and ½ of a grapefruit (low-sugar fruit)
Snack: DWL and 1 cup of whole strawberries (low-sugar fruit)	**Snack:** DWL product
Dinner: Grilled wild salmon (quality protein) with mashed cauliflower (low-sugar vegetable)	**Dinner:** Steak (quality protein) with asparagus (low-sugar vegetable)
Dessert: DWL product	**Dessert:** DWL product

DAY 11

Breakfast: 2 eggs (2 ounces of quality protein) and ½ cup raspberries (low-sugar fruit)

Snack: DWL product

Lunch: DWL product plus 1 cup of your favorite green vegetables (low-sugar vegetable)

Snack: DWL product

Dinner: Mexican Platter—grilled chicken (4 ounces quality protein), black beans (2 ounces quality protein) topped with grated cheese, shredded cabbage (low-sugar vegetable), sliced avocado, and dollop of Greek yogurt (healthy fats), and salsa

Dessert: DWL product

DAY 12

Breakfast: DWL product

Snack: Greek yogurt (healthy fat) topped with blueberries (low-sugar fruit)

Lunch: DWL product plus side salad (low-sugar vegetable)

Snack: DWL product

Dinner: Grilled turkey burger (quality protein) and side of broccoli (low-sugar vegetable)

Dessert: DWL product

DAY 13

Breakfast: DWL product and two apricots (low-sugar fruit)

Snack: Handful of raw walnuts (healthy fat)

Lunch: DWL product and side of Brussels sprouts (low-sugar vegetable)

Snack: DWL product

Dinner: Spaghetti squash "pasta" with meat sauce

Dessert: DWL product

DAY 14

Breakfast: DWL product

Snack: Celery sticks (low-carb vegetable) dipped in hummus (2 ounces of protein)

Lunch: DWL product

Snack: DWL product

Dinner: Grilled boneless pork chops (quality protein), asparagus (low-sugar vegetable), and sliced avocado (healthy fat)

Dessert: DWL product

DAY 15

Breakfast: Three-egg (protein) omelet with spinach (vegetable) and cheese (fat), with a side of blueberries (fruit)

Snack: DWL product

Lunch: DWL product

Snack: DWL product

Dinner: DWL product

DAY 16

Breakfast: DWL product

Snack: DWL product

Lunch: Bun-less burger (protein) topped with cheese (fat), lettuce/tomato/onion (vegetable and fruit), and optional low-sugar ketchup and/or mustard

Snack: DWL product

Dinner: DWL product

DAY 17	DAY 18
Breakfast: Cottage cheese (protein) with strawberries (fruit)	**Breakfast:** DWL product
Snack: DWL product	**Snack:** DWL product
Lunch: DWL product with salad (vegetable) topped with avocado (fat)	**Lunch:** Bed of greens (vegetable) topped with canned tuna (protein), mixed with mayonnaise (fat), diced onions and bell peppers (fruit), and chopped celery (vegetable)
Snack: DWL product	
Dinner: DWL product with side of roasted broccoli (vegetable)	**Snack:** DWL product
	Dinner: DWL product

DAY 19	DAY 20
Breakfast: Sliced cucumbers (fruit) topped with cream cheese (fat) and smoked salmon (protein)	**Breakfast:** DWL product
	Snack: DWL product
Snack: DWL product	**Lunch:** Lettuce cups (vegetable) filled with deli turkey slices (protein), avocado (fat), scallion, and optional mayonnaise and/or mustard
Lunch: DWL product	
Snack: DWL product	
Dinner: DWL product with a side of grilled asparagus (vegetable)	**Snack:** DWL product
	Dinner: DWL product with a side of roasted Brussels sprouts (vegetable)

DAY 21	
Breakfast: Low-sugar yogurt (protein) topped with strawberries (fruit) and crushed walnuts (fat)	
Snack: DWL product	
Lunch: DWL product with a side salad (vegetable)	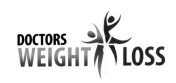
Snack: DWL product	
Dinner: DWL product with a side of Parmesan-topped roasted cauliflower (vegetable)	

CHAPTER 8
Doctors Weight Loss Lifestyle Plan

The Doctors Weight Loss Lifestyle Plan is for someone who has been adhering to the accelerated plan (found in the previous chapter) and who has come within five pounds of their goal weight, or it's for someone who is just starting their weight loss journey but prefers a fairly even balance of medical-grade weight loss products to standard grocery fare. First of all, you need 90 units of medical-grade weight loss products which will allow three prepackaged products per day, along with two sensible meals consisting of vegetables, proteins, an optional healthy fat, and an optional low-sugar fruit. When ordering your products at doctorsweightloss.com keep in mind that most boxes contain seven units of products, however, a handful contain only five units. If you're ordering all boxes with seven units, you'll need (roughly) thirteen boxes of products, but remember to adjust accordingly if you order a five-unit box.

The Lifestyle Plan can be adhered to until you have reached your goal weight or it can be used as a stepping-stone from the accelerated and life-style plans as a wean-off system to go from medical-grade products to all standard foods. The following chapter will show you how to incorporate even more foods and one less product while still achieving and maintaining your weight loss goals. The two to three servings of vegetables, ten to fourteen ounces of protein, one optional healthy fat, and one optional low-sugar fruit can be eaten within two meals, or spread out through the day however you desire.

Below you will find a sample visual meal plan which follows this plan's guidelines. Three of the photos are of the actual Doctors Weight Loss (DWL) medical-grade products and you will see they look (and taste) just like your old favorites. Two of the photos are of the sensible meals you will be responsible for preparing—those meals incorporate the protein, vegetables, and optional heathy fat and fruit. Further into this chapter, you will find a sample seven-day lifestyle meal plan.

Lifestyle Plan Allowance per Day

2–3 Medical-grade weight loss products
2–3 servings low-carbohydrate vegetables
1 serving low-sugar fruit (optional)
1 serving healthy fat (optional)
10–14 ounces quality protein

Lifestyle Meal Plan One

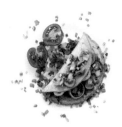
Sensible meal

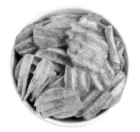
DWL high-protein chips

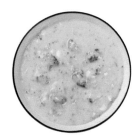
DWL high-protein soup

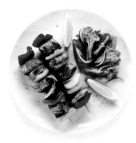
Sensible meal

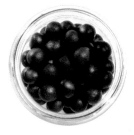
DWL high-protein chocolates

Lifestyle Meal Plan Two

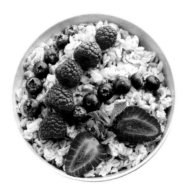

DWL high-protein oatmeal

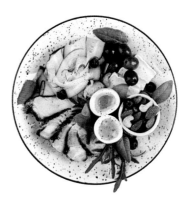

Sensible meal

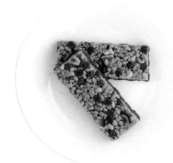

DWL high-protein bar

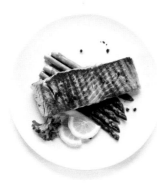

Sensible meal

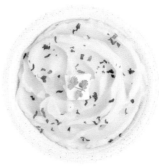

DWL high-protein mashed potatoes

Now let's put all of these guidelines in place to exhibit a typical one-week lifestyle meal plan.

DAY 1	DAY 2
Breakfast: DWL product	**Breakfast:** DWL product
Snack: DWL product	**Snack:** Serving of raspberries
Lunch: Canned tuna (quality protein) with mustard and extra-virgin olive oil (fat) served with celery stick (vegetable) dippers	**Lunch:** Lettuce cups (vegetable) with sliced deli meat (protein), avocado (fat), and mustard
Snack: DWL product	**Snack:** DWL product
Dinner: Grilled chicken breast (protein) with roasted Brussels sprouts (vegetable)	**Dinner:** Grilled wild salmon (protein) with broccoli (vegetable)
	Dessert: DWL product
DAY 3	**DAY 4**
Breakfast: DWL product	**Breakfast:** Cottage cheese (protein) topped with blueberries (fruit)
Snack: Serving of strawberries (fruit)	**Snack:** DWL product
Lunch: Bed of raw spinach (vegetable) topped with chicken (protein), goat cheese and crushed walnuts (fat), and low-carb salad dressing	**Lunch:** Two hardboiled eggs mixed with mayonnaise (protein and fat) with celery sticks (vegetable) to dip
Snack: DWL product	**Snack:** DWL product
Dinner: Steak (protein) with a steamed artichoke (vegetable)	**Dinner:** Chopped chicken (protein) cooked in salsa verde, with grated cheese/sour cream/mashed avocado (fat) and shredded cabbage (vegetable)
Dessert: DWL product	**Dessert:** DWL product

DAY 5	DAY 6
Breakfast: DWL product	**Breakfast:** DWL product
Snack: Piece of cheese (fat)	**Snack:** Broccoli florets (vegetable) dipped in hummus (protein)
Lunch: DWL product	**Lunch:** Chicken and vegetable soup (protein and vegetable)
Dinner: Grilled turkey burger (protein) with side of green beans (vegetable); optional turkey burger add-ons include mustard, low-sugar ketchup, cheese, avocado, tomato, and onion	**Snack:** DWL product
	Dinner: Spaghetti squash "pasta" (fruit) topped with meat sauce (protein), and a side of Brussels sprouts (vegetable)
Dessert: DWL product	**Dessert:** DWL product
DAY 7	
Breakfast: DWL product	
Snack: Serving of raspberries	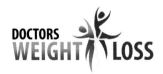
Lunch: DWL product	
Dinner: Grilled boneless pork chops (protein), asparagus (vegetable), and sauerkraut (vegetable)	
Dessert: DWL product	

CHAPTER 9

Doctors Weight Loss Maintenance Plan

The Doctors Weight Loss Maintenance Plan is for someone who has been adhering to the accelerated and/or lifestyle plans and who has come within five pounds of their goal weight, or it's for someone who is just starting their weight loss journey but prefers mostly standard grocery fare with just two medical-grade products per day to use as high-protein snacks when on-the-go. First of all, you need 60 units of medical-grade weight loss products which will allow two prepackaged products per day for one month, along with three sensible meals consisting of vegetables, proteins, an optional healthy fat, and an optional low-sugar fruit. When ordering your products at doctorsweightloss.com keep in mind that most boxes contain seven units of products, however, a handful contain only five units. If you're ordering all boxes with seven units, you'll need (roughly) thirteen boxes of products, but remember to adjust accordingly if you order a five-unit box.

The Maintenance Plan can be followed until you have reached your goal weight or it can be used as a stepping-stone from the accelerated and lifestyle plans as a wean-off system to go from medical-grade

Maintenance Plan Allowance per Day

1–2 medical-grade weight loss products

2–3 servings low-carbohydrate vegetables

1 serving low-sugar fruit (optional)

1 serving healthy fat (optional)

12–18 ounces quality protein

products to all standard foods. The following chapter will show you how to adopt your new low-carb lifestyle using only grocery foods, without the assistance from medical-grade weight loss products. The two to three servings of vegetables, twelve to eighteen ounces of protein, one optional healthy fat, and one optional low-sugar fruit can be eaten within three meals, or spread out through the day however you desire.

Below you will find a sample visual meal plan which follows the above-mentioned guidelines. Two of the photos are of the actual Doctors Weight Loss (DWL) medical-grade products and you will see they look (and taste) just like your old favorites. Three of the photos are of the sensible meals you will be responsible for preparing—those meals incorporate the protein, vegetables, and optional heathy fat and fruit. Further into this chapter, you will find a sample seven-day maintenance meal plan.

Sample Maintenance Plan One

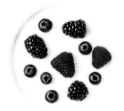

Sensible meal

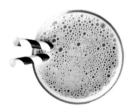

DWL high-protein shake

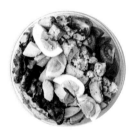

Sensible meal

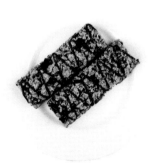

DWL high-protein bar

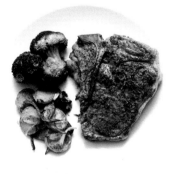

Sensible meal

Now let's put all of these guidelines in place to exhibit a typical one-week accelerated meal plan.

DAY 1	DAY 2
Breakfast: Two or three eggs (protein) cooked your way with a side of berries	**Breakfast:** Greek yogurt (protein) topped with berries (fruit)
Snack: DWL product	**Snack:** DWL product
Lunch: Canned tuna (protein) mixed with mustard and extra-virgin olive oil (fat) with celery sticks (vegetable) to dip	**Lunch:** Lettuce cups (vegetable) filled with deli sliced turkey (protein) and your favorite sandwich additions
Snack: DWL product	**Dinner:** Grilled salmon (protein) with broccoli (vegetable)
Dinner: Grilled chicken breast (protein) with Brussels sprouts (vegetable)	**Dessert:** DWL product
DAY 3	DAY 4
Breakfast: Protein oatmeal (using ¼ cup dry rolled oats, cook on stovetop with half amount of water you would normally use, and with two eggs whites (protein); cook all of the way through according to directions and top with blueberries (fruit))	**Breakfast:** Sliced cucumbers (fruit) topped with cream cheese (fat) and smoked salmon (protein)
Snack: DWL product	**Snack:** DWL product
Lunch: Bed of leafy greens (vegetable) topped with roasted or canned chicken (protein), avocado (fat), and low-carb salad dressing	**Lunch:** Burger with no bun topped with lettuce, tomato, and onion, low-sugar ketchup and mustard, with a side of broccoli (vegetable)
Snack: DWL product	**Snack:** DWL product
Dinner: Steak (protein) with a steamed artichoke (vegetable)	**Dinner:** Chopped chicken (protein) sautéed in green tomatillo sauce with optional toppings of shredded cheese, sliced avocado, sour cream, onions, tomato, cilantro, and salsa

DAY 5	DAY 6
Breakfast: Avocado shake (blend ¼ cup plain yogurt (protein), 2 splashes of milk or nondairy creamer, ½ an avocado (fat), ½ cup blueberries (fruit), and ice; add a drizzle of honey or zero-calorie sweetener if desired)	**Breakfast:** Cottage cheese (protein) topped with strawberries (fruit)
	Snack: DWL product
Snack: DWL product	**Lunch:** Avocado (fat) stuffed with bay shrimp (protein) and topped with cocktail or hot sauce
Lunch: Chicken (protein) and vegetable soup (no noodles or rice) with a side salad (vegetable)	**Snack:** DWL product
Dinner: Roasted turkey (protein) and a side of steamed cauliflower (vegetable) mashed with Parmesan cheese	**Dinner:** Cod (protein) with one portion of roasted sweet potato, and a side salad (vegetable)
Dessert: DWL product	

DAY 7	
Breakfast: On-the-go breakfast snack pack: one hard-boiled egg (protein), plain yogurt (protein), topped with blueberries (fruit), and a serving of nuts (fat)	
Snack: DWL product	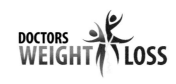
Lunch: Baked chicken wings (protein) with a side of celery (vegetable) and low-carb dipping sauce	
Snack: DWL product	
Dinner: Pork chops (protein), asparagus (vegetable), and sauerkraut	

CHAPTER 10

The Fastest and Easiest Way to Start Your New Low-Carb Life

An easy start-up process is key to starting any nutrition plan. The preparation to begin some food plans is so daunting that many put off beginning in the first place! Keep in mind, we have many meal plans, recipes, meal preparation tactics, and unique low-carb foods to choose from so days to come will be far more varied, with the option to whip up interesting recipes. People are most likely to start a new regimen if it's easy, and that means not dealing with unfamiliar or hard-to-find foods, long preparation times, or expensive kitchen gadgets. The Low-Carb Meal Planning Kit is the easiest formula to implement for formatting your meals. We urge you to use this kit for at least a week to learn the ropes of low-carb meal planning. If you stick to it only for the first seven days, you will see results on the scale that fast! And if you decide to continue with this meal planning system indefinitely, that is perfectly fine.

For meal examples that employ this chart, you will find five breakfast, five lunch, five dinner, and five snack options—they are all low-carb-approved so the guesswork is taken out for you, and you'll be on your way to your weight loss and wellness goals! For the next few days, pick a breakfast, lunch, dinner, and one or two snacks from the list on the following pages, or create your own meals using the chart to the right.

LOW-CARB MEAL PLANNING KIT				
Pick a protein	Pick a low-carb produce or two	Add a fat or two	Pick one serving of low-sugar fruit per day (optional)	Optional condiments for any meal
Chicken	Cauliflower	Olive oil	Raspberries	Mustard
Steak	Broccoli	Avocado oil	Strawberries	Sugar-free seasonings
Ground beef	Broccoli rabe	Coconut oil	Blackberries	Hot sauce
Fish	Swiss chard	Walnut oil	Blueberries	Freshly squeezed lemon/lime
Shellfish	Zucchini	MCT oil		Fresh or dried herbs and spices
Pork	Spaghetti squash	Grass-fed butter		Vinegar
Turkey	Mushrooms	Grass-fed ghee		
Ground turkey	Asparagus	Cheese		
Lamb	Brussels sprouts	Bacon		
Venison	Leafy greens/ side salad	Avocado		
Plant-based protein (low-carb, low-sugar)	Spinach	High-fat, low-carb, low-sugar sauce or dressing		
Dairy-based protein (cottage cheese, Greek yogurt, kefir)	Onion (no more than two tablespoons per serving, due to carb content)	Nuts/seeds Nut/seed butters		
Eggs	Cabbage	Eggs		
	Green beans	Olives		
	Cucumber	Avocado oil mayonnaise		
	Tomato	Regular mayonnaise		
	Bell pepper	Coconut milk		
	Eggplant	Cream		

Breakfast Options
Choose One

2–3 eggs cooked in oil your way, topped with cheese (optional) and avocado (optional) with side of berries or sliced tomatoes.

2–3 egg omelet with sautéed onions, bell peppers, and mushrooms, topped with cheese (optional) and avocado (optional).

2–3 eggs your way with 1–2 pieces of bacon.

Plain Greek yogurt or nondairy yogurt topped with berries and nuts or seeds.

Cottage cheese with berries or tomatoes.

Breakfast box to-go: 1 hard-boiled egg, 1 string cheese, 2–3 ounces smoked salmon, sliced avocado, handful favorite berries.

Lunch Options
Choose One

Green salad topped with chicken or steak, shredded cheese, sliced avocado, olives, oil and vinegar or store-bought ranch or blue cheese dressing (no sugar added).

1–2 cans of tuna or chicken mixed with mayonnaise, mustard, diced celery, and diced red onion. Eat on its own or use celery sticks to dip.

Deli sandwich lettuce wrap: fill one or two large iceberg lettuce cups with your favorite deli meats and cheeses, and any or all of the following: mayonnaise, mustard, avocado, tomato, onion, pickle.

Turkey burger or hamburger with no bun, topped with any or all of the following toppings: cheese, mayonnaise, mustard, avocado, tomato, onion, pickle.

Protein platter: chicken, steak, or fish prepared with any of the following: melted cheese, sliced avocado, sautéed green vegetables, sauerkraut, green salad with oil and vinegar.

Dinner Options
Choose One

Sliced chicken, onion, and bell pepper sautéed in oil and store-bought tomatillo sauce (green sauce). Top with shredded cheese, sour cream, mashed avocado, and cilantro.

Steak topped with butter, paired with sautéed or roasted asparagus, and small side salad topped with oil and vinegar.

Salmon (or other fish) pan-cooked in grass-fed butter or ghee, paired with steamed cauliflower mashed with Parmesan cheese.

Hamburger (no bun) topped with cheese, mayonnaise, mustard, lettuce, tomato, onion, and avocado paired with green vegetable of choice.

Lamb chops or lamb steak topped with tzatziki (combine Greek yogurt, garlic, diced cucumber, and freshly squeezed lemon) paired with green vegetable of choice.

Low-Carb Snacks (pick one or two per day)

Serving of nuts or seeds.
Piece of cheese.
Beef jerky.
Celery dipped in nut butter or cream cheese.
Red bell pepper slices with cream cheese and
"Everything but the Bagel" seasoning.
Hard-boiled egg.
2–3 squares dark chocolate (at least 75 percent cacao).
Serving of olives.
Serving of berries.
Sliced tomatoes drizzled with olive oil and seasonings.
Half avocado with melted cheese and salsa.
Jicama or endive leave dipped in mashed avocado.
Sliced cucumber dipped in ranch dressing.
Celery dipped in blue cheese dressing.
Salami slices with cream cheese and sliced pickles.
Deli turkey or ham rolled up with a piece of cheese.
Coconut cream or half-and-half with raspberries.

You can repeat meals if you like—for example, if you already have some eggs in the fridge and that means less grocery shopping, have eggs for breakfast each day. Or if you want to make the tuna/chicken salad ahead of time and have it both days, that is fine too. We want to make the adjustment to your new nutrition plan as easy and inexpensive as possible. If this type of simplistic meal planning works for you (as it does for many!), you can use this system for as long as you like, as these foods make up a solid foundation of the low-carb diet. If you want something new and more varied, keep on reading to further chapters!

Food	Calories	Visual Cue
Vegetables		
1 cup green vegetables	25 calories	1 baseball
2 cups leafy greens (raw)	25 calories	2 baseballs
Low-Sugar Fruits		
½ cup berries	45 calories	1 tennis ball
½ cup sliced tomato	15 calories	1 tennis ball
½ cup sliced bell pepper	15 calories	1 tennis ball
Fats		
½ cup sliced avocado	115 calories	1 tennis ball
1 tablespoon oil	120 calories	3 dice
1 tablespoon butter	100 calories	3 dice
1 tablespoon ghee	135 calories	3 dice
1 tablespoon mayonnaise	103 calories	3 dice
6 ounces salmon	300 calories	2 decks of cards
1 ounce nuts	160–205 calories	2 golf balls
2 tablespoons nut/seed butter	95–175 calories	1 golf ball
1 cup full-fat yogurt	150 calories	1 baseball
1 cup full-fat cottage cheese	200 calories	1 baseball
1 ounce olives	60 calories	10 whole olives
Proteins		
6 ounces chicken/turkey	200–275 calories	2 decks of cards
6 ounces steak	320 calories	2 decks of cards
6 ounces fish	150–310 calories	2 decks of cards
6 ounces shellfish	130–170 calories	2 handfuls
6 ounces ground beef	360 calories	2 decks of cards

Portions and Serving Sizes

We do not want you to count calories and weigh foods religiously—essentially, if you stick to the plans in this book, your low-carb macros will fall into place. To the left is a portion guide to help you gauge a sensible portion that is most effective for results. Of course, this is a simplified list of low-carb foods—if you would like to see everything you can eat, refer back to chapter 5.

Beverages

As with food, we need to stick to zero-sugar and/or extremely low sugar beverages. Water is always your best bet, however, unsweetened coffee and tea with dairy- or nondairy creamer is low-carb-approved. In addition, unsweetened sparkling water and bone broth are allowed, as well as one or two glasses of low sugar wine (per day) such as cabernet sauvignon, merlot, pinot noir, chardonnay, pinot grigio, and sauvignon blanc with dinner. Rum, whiskey, tequila, vodka, and gin are all low-carb-friendly, however, they cannot be combined with sugary mixers.

Congratulations for embarking on your low-carb journey. Remember to weigh yourself the morning of your first official day of food, as you will probably see results after even the first seventy-two hours. Keep in mind, although this low-carb meal planning kit and basic guidelines found in this chapter are simple, it is the foundation for the low-carb lifestyle. If you choose to keep using this system for longer than a few days, feel free—it works! You will be given more meal plans, recipes, and interesting ways to whip up delicious and unique fare in coming chapters.

CHAPTER 11

The Low-Carb Seven-Day Meal Plan Photo Guide

This seven-day meal plan is not only easy to put together, you can also find all of these ingredients in most mainstream grocery stores. There are no recipes or measurements as this meal plan requires you to only put simple foods together with minimal preparation. If you are unsure of how to prepare each meal or snack, refer to the photo as an easy reference. As a reminder of food serving sizes, you can refer back to page 76.

✳ ✳ ✳

Breakfast: Cottage cheese topped with berries and nuts

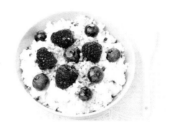

Snack: Celery with peanut butter

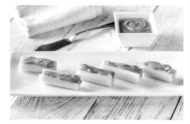

Lunch: Deli meat lettuce wrap

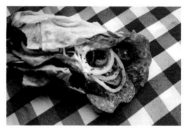

Snack: Serving of pork rinds

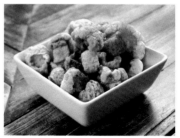

Dinner: Halibut with spinach and leeks

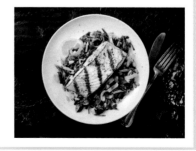

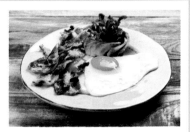

Breakfast: Traditional bacon and eggs with sliced avocado

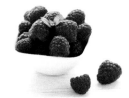

Snack: Serving of raspberries

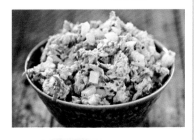

Lunch: Tuna salad

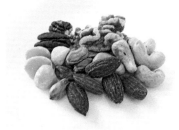

Snack: Serving of nuts

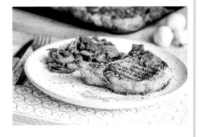

Dinner: Pork chop with sautéed spinach and mushrooms

Breakfast: Cucumber slices with cream cheese and smoked salmon

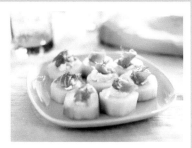

Snack: Hard-boiled egg

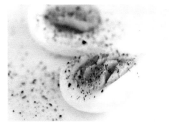

Lunch: Hamburger (no bun) with toppings

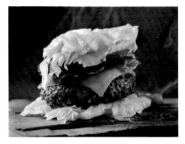

Snack: Piece of cheese

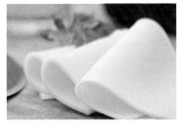

Dinner: Chicken with avocado salsa

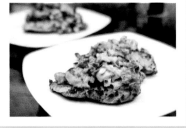

Breakfast: Spinach and cheese omelet with tomatoes

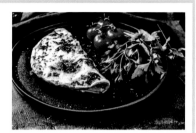

Snack: Serving of olives

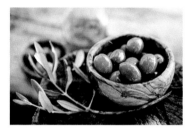

Lunch: Chicken wings with celery sticks and blue cheese dressing

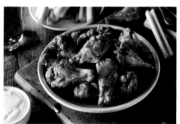

Snack: Serving of nuts

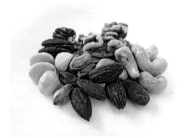

Dinner: Salmon with asparagus

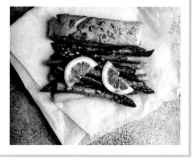

Breakfast: Plain yogurt topped with strawberries and walnuts

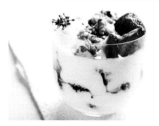

Snack: High-fat coffee with coconut oil and butter

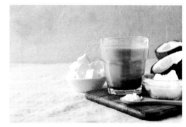

Lunch: Ground turkey in endive leaves topped with guacamole

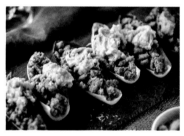

Snack: Deli meat wrapped string cheese

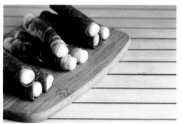

Dinner: Lamb chops with a side salad

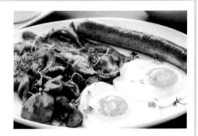

Breakfast: Eggs, sausage, bacon, mushroom, and tomato platter

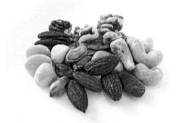

Snack: Serving of nuts

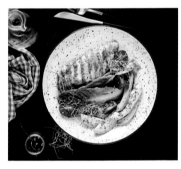

Lunch: Chicken and avocado salad

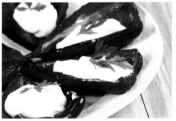

Snack: Bell pepper and cream cheese

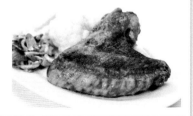

Dinner: Roasted turkey (skin on) with mashed cauliflower

Breakfast: Smoked salmon, egg, asparagus, nuts, and cheese bento box

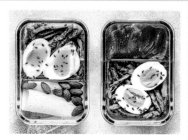

Snack: Cottage cheese topped with berries and nuts

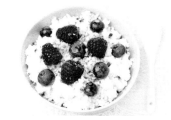

Lunch: Shrimp and avocado salad

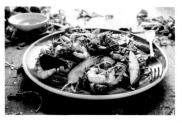

Snack: Serving of nuts

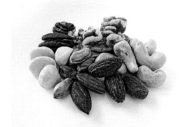

Dinner: Rib eye with green vegetables

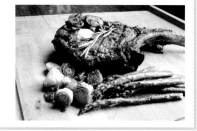

If you prefer some meals and snacks over others, choose your favorites and feel free to have some repetition—that will also cut down on grocery shopping time when you have less variety. Also, eating five times per day (three meals and two snacks) is not required. Only eat if you feel hungry, so if you're content with less meals and/or snacks, feel free to adjust this plan as needed.

CHAPTER 12
Low-Carb Food Groups and Servings

If you're the type of nutrition planner who wants to know exact servings and amounts to eat, this chapter is for you. The types of calories you consume are just as (if not more) important than the amounts of calories you consume. Due to their macro- and micronutrient contents, the following food groups are essential for weight loss, steady blood sugar levels, and overall wellbeing, so we highly recommend making these guidelines an everyday goal to fulfill. It is important to note that you are *not* restricted to the foods listed on the next few pages; these food groups should take priority in your daily low-carb regimen, however, you will be able to incorporate other foods as well. For the complete list of acceptable low-carb foods, please refer back to chapter 5.

① Low-Glycemic Vegetables (2–3 servings or more)

Nutrient-dense vegetables are a good source of low-glycemic carbohydrates that will give you energy but help maintain even blood sugar levels. Several vitamins, such as vitamins A and C, and minerals such as iron and magnesium, are also found in these vegetables; plus many are high in calcium and fiber! If you do not see your favorite low-glycemic vegetable below, feel free to include it in your daily food regimen. The average amount of calories, carbohydrates, protein, fat, and fiber for the vegetables we provided are 12 calories, 2 grams of carbohydrates, 1 gram of protein, 0 grams of fat, and 2 grams of fiber in case you would like to compare your vegetable of choice to the ones in the recommended list.

Green Vegetable	Serving Size	Calories	Carbohydrates	Protein	Fat	Fiber
Spinach (cooked)	½ cup	23	4g	3g	0g	2.5g
Broccoli	½ cup	16	3g	1.5g	0g	1g
Kale	½ cup	17	3g	1.5g	0g	1g
Collard greens	½ cup	6	1g	0.5g	0g	0.5g
Cabbage	½ cup	9	2g	0.5g	0g	1g
Brussels sprouts	½ cup	19	4g	1.5g	0g	1.5g
Bok choy	½ cup	5	1g	0.5g	0g	0g
Romaine lettuce	½ cup	8	0.5g	0.5g	0g	0g
Arugula	½ cup	3	0g	0g	0g	0g
Cauliflower	½ cup	13	2.5g	1g	0g	1g

The number of servings of low-glycemic vegetables you eat per day will be based on your personal caloric needs. Since everyone is different, you can tailor your green vegetable needs based on your overall caloric intake requirements, as well as the low-carb macronutrient percentages you are targeting each day, given the amount of other consumed foods.

② Low-Sugar Nonfatty Fruits (0–2 serving)

Low-sugar fruits are another source of carbohydrates and energy. In addition, they provide even more micronutrients to add to the variety of benefits the low-glycemic vegetables boast. Try to incorporate tomato or red bell pepper in your servings of low-sugar fruits as they contain lycopene, which is a powerful antioxidant that is beneficial for heart health, sun protection, and reduced risk of certain cancers. Do not have more than one serving of berries per day in order to stick to your carbohydrate requirements. Please stick to the following low-glycemic fruit choices, as the selections we have hand-picked for you are the lowest in sugar, and remaining extremely low in sugar will be most advantageous for reaching your goals. The average amount of calories, carbohydrates, protein, fat, and fiber for the fruits we provided are 27 calories, 6½ grams of carbohydrates, 1 gram of protein, 0 grams of fat, and 2 grams of fiber.

Low-Sugar Fruit	Serving Size	Calories	Carbohydrates	Protein	Fat	Fiber
Tomato	½ cup	16	3.5g	1g	0g	1g
Bell pepper	½ cup	15	3.5g	0g	0g	1g
Blueberries	½ cup	43	11g	0.5g	0g	2g
Raspberries	½ cup	33	8g	1g	0g	4g
Strawberries	½ cup	25	6g	0.5g	0g	1.5g
Blackberries	½ cup	31	7g	1g	0g	4g

The number of servings of low-sugar fruits you eat per day will be based on your personal caloric needs. Since everyone is different, you can tailor your low-sugar fruit needs based on your overall caloric intake requirements.

(3) Summer and Winter Squash (0–1 serving)

Squash is mistakenly known as a vegetable or tuber but it's actually a fruit, and it is another source of carbohydrates that contain essential nutrients and antioxidants. Since this protocol requires us to remain extremely low in carbohydrates and sugar, it is important to note the lower-carbohydrate variety of squash, which is the summer squash (zucchini, zephyr, and cousa) however, zephyr and cousa can be hard to find in some grocery stores. Up to two servings per day are allowed for these varieties and up to one serving per day is allowed of the winter varieties (butternut squash, pumpkin, spaghetti squash, and acorn squash). Please stick to the choices below as other starches are too high in carbohydrates for the typical low-carb regimen. The average amount of calories, carbohydrates, protein, fat, and fiber for the starches we provided are 24 calories, 6 grams of carbohydrates, 1 gram of protein, 0 grams of fat, and 1 gram of fiber.

Squash Fruits	Serving Size	Calories	Carbohydrates	Protein	Fat	Fiber
Zucchini	1 cup	21	4g	1.5g	0.5g	1g
Zephyr	1 cup	19	4g	1.5g	0g	1g
Cousa	1 cup	20	4g	1.5g	0.5g	1g
Butternut squash	½ cup	32	8g	1g	0g	1.5g
Pumpkin	½ cup	15	4g	0.5g	0g	0g
Spaghetti squash	1 cup	31	7g	1g	1g	1.5g
Acorn squash	½ cup	28	8g	0.5g	0g	1g

Whether you eat zero or one serving of squash per day will be based on your personal caloric needs, as well as the amount of other carbohydrates you have eaten or will plan to eat on the same day. Since everyone is different, you can tailor your squash needs based on your overall caloric intake requirements.

④ Protein (3–5 servings)

Protein contains amino acids, which are the essential building blocks of muscle, which burns fat, but not all proteins are created equal. It is imperative to consume high-quality proteins (organic, grass-fed, and wild if possible) that are unprocessed and have minimal preservatives, fillers, and environmental toxins. If you do not see your favorite protein below, feel free to include it in your daily food regimen. The average amount of calories, carbohydrates, protein, fat, and fiber for the proteins we provided are 116 calories, ½ gram of carbohydrates, 19 grams of protein, 4 grams of fat, and 0 grams of fiber in case you would like to compare your protein choice to the ones in the recommended list.

Protein	Serving Size	Calories	Carbohydrates	Protein	Fat	Fiber
Eggs	1 large egg	78	0.5g	6g	5g	0g
Chicken (boneless, skinless)	3 ounces	90	0g	17g	1.5g	0g
Turkey (boneless, skinless)	3 ounces	120	0g	26g	1g	0g
Cod	3 ounces	70	0g	15g	1g	0g
Shrimp	3 ounces	90	1g	17g	1.5g	0g
Scallops	3 ounces	90	5g	17g	0.5g	0g
Wild salmon	3 ounces	143	0g	18g	8g	0g
Lean beef	3 ounces	158	0g	26g	5g	0g
Chicken with skin	3 ounces	190	0g	20g	11g	0g
Turkey with skin	3 ounces	129	0g	24g	3g	0g
Canned Tuna (packed in water)	3 ounces	90	0g	20g	1g	0g
Boneless pork chops	3 ounces	115	0g	20g	4g	0g
Bone-in pork chops	3 ounces	150	0g	17g	7g	0g

The number of servings of protein you eat per day will be based on your personal caloric needs. Since everyone is different, you can tailor your protein needs based on your overall caloric intake requirements. If you add your own protein to the list, be sure to avoid low-quality choices that have detrimental additives such as nitrates; items such as hot dogs, deli meats, and fast-food meats should be eliminated or severely limited.

(5) Fats (2–3 servings)

This group contains the beneficial fats that include properties that assist with weight loss, increasing good cholesterol, reducing bad cholesterol, and maintaining even blood sugar levels. The average amount of calories, carbohydrates, protein, fat, and fiber for the healthy fats below are 116 calories, 1½ grams of carbohydrates, 5 grams of protein, 11 grams of fat, and 1 gram of fiber.

Fatty Food	Serving Size	Calories	Carbohydrates	Protein	Fat	Fiber
Avocado	½ cup	117	6g	1.5g	11g	5g
Walnuts	14 halves	185	4g	4g	18g	2g
Wild salmon	3 ounces	143	0g	18g	8g	0g
Eggs	1 large egg	78	0.5g	6g	5g	0g
Extra-virgin olive oil	1 tablespoon	119	0g	0g	14g	0g
Coconut oil	1 tablespoon	121	0g	0g	14g	0g
Avocado oil	1 tablespoon	124	0g	0g	14g	0g
Macadamia nuts	1 ounce	204	4g	2g	21g	2.5g
Brazil nuts	1 ounce	186	3.5g	4g	19g	2g
Fatty cuts of meat	3 ounces	158	0g	26g	15g	0g
Cream	1 tablespoon	29	0.5g	0.5g	3g	0g
Coconut milk	2 tablespoons	68	2g	1g	7g	1g
Olives	1 ounce	41	1g	0g	4g	1g
Cheddar cheese	1 ounce	113	0.5g	7g	9g	0g
Mozzarella cheese	1 ounce	78	1g	8g	5g	0g
Cottage cheese	½ cup	111	4g	12g	5g	0g
Grass-fed butter	1 tablespoon	100	0g	0g	11g	0g

The number of servings of fats you eat per day will be based on your personal caloric needs, as well as the amounts of macronutrients consumed from other foods. Since everyone is different, you can tailor your healthy fat needs based on your overall caloric intake requirements.

If you're unsure of how to incorporate these foods into a meal plan, the Low-Carb Select Meal Planning System found in chapter 13 will detail a variety of ways to meet the above recommended requirements. For the most simplistic way to achieve these servings, you can also refer back to chapter 4's Low-Carb Meal Planning Kit. If you want to get even more creative, the breakfast, lunch, and dinner recipes found in chapter 19, 20, and 21 include a variety of these foods, incorporated into delicious meals.

CHAPTER 13
The Low-Carb Select Meal Planning System

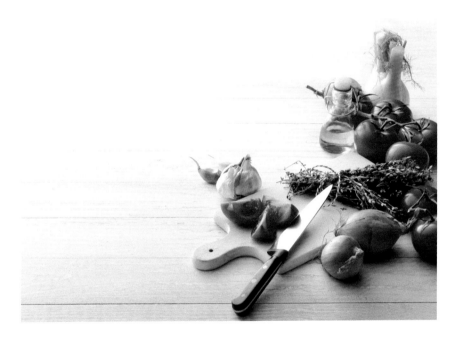

The Low-Carb Select Meal Planning System is your simplistic guide to daily food recommendations that can be used when you need quick and easy ideas for breakfast, lunch, dinner, and snacks. You will be given different categories to select from which will lead to the proper low-carb and high-protein macros on your plate. You may be wondering, *Do I use the Low-Carb Select Meal Planning System or the recipes found in coming chapters?* The meal planning system found in this chapter is a road map of basic food choices to follow and it's specifically designed for those who don't have time for recipes. If you find yourself on a lazy Sunday where you do have some time to experiment, feel free to try the more complex breakfast, lunch, and dinner recipes found in the following recipes chapters.

Unlike the typical, rigid meal plan, the low-carb select meal planning system gives you several options for breakfast, lunch, dinner, and snacks—it's a "choose your own adventure" of sorts. At the beginning of each section (breakfast, lunch, dinner, beverages, snacks), you will be given a set of directions which will explain possible food options for that particular meal or snack. This will allow for some flexibility with regard to your taste buds, how hungry you are, caloric needs, and what you have in the pantry or refrigerator. The Low-Carb Select Meal Planning System is based on simplicity, convenience, and foods that are sound with regard to overall health, as well as weight loss. If you are feeling more adventurous, feel free to substitute any meal with one of the delicious recipes found in chapters 19, 20, and 21. Or you can even create your own unique daily food plans using the breakfast, lunch, and dinner recipes found in those chapters as all meals exhibited provide dense nutrition, while following the guidelines of the low-carb nutrition plan.

The items listed in the meal planning system are easily found in most grocery stores and the majority of the instructions (we won't even call them recipes) are easy, not calling for too many ingredients or too much preparation. We do not list every single low-carb-approved food in the meal planning system, so if you're wondering about appropriate substitutions, refer back to chapter 5 to make sure your food is allowed on your plan. If you're unsure of the appropriate serving size, the nutrition label of a particular food will list how much of the item should be consumed for one serving or you can refer the serving size chart found on page 76.

How to Meal Plan—Breakfast

Choose one or two options from the protein category, one or two from the fat category, and one or two selections from the low-glycemic produce category. If you select two from the low-glycemic produce section, no more than one can come from berries.

Protein

One, Two, or Three Eggs Your Way: Choose your favorite preparation style—boiled, poached, scrambled, over easy, or sunny-side up.

One or Two Eggs Your Way with Smoked Salmon, Bacon, or Sausage: Choose your favorite egg preparation style and pair with two to three ounces of smoked salmon, two to three slices of uncured, nitrate-free bacon, or two to three pieces of breakfast sausage.

Smoked Salmon: 3–4 ounces
Herring: 3–4 ounces
Bacon: 2–3 pieces
Breakfast Sausage: 2–4 ounces
Steak: 4–8 ounces
Cheese: 1–2 ounces
Cottage Cheese: ½–1 cup
Plain Yogurt, Kefir, or Nondairy Yogurt: ½–⅔ cup

Low-Glycemic Produce

Strawberries: 4–5 medium
Blueberries: ½ cup
Raspberries: ½ cup
Blackberries: ½ cup
Mixed berries: ½ cup
Tomato: ½ cup, sliced
Avocado: ½, sliced or mashed
Bell pepper: ½ cup, sliced or diced
Mushrooms: ½ cup, sliced or diced
Onions: ¼ cup, sliced or diced
Spinach: 1 cup raw or ½ cup cooked
Kale: 1 cup raw or ½ cup cooked
Asparagus: 2–3 spears
Broccoli: ½–1 cup, cooked
Leafy greens: 1–2 cups
Omelet Produce Mix (onions, bell pepper, mushrooms): ½ cup

Fat

Avocado: ½, sliced or mashed

Olives: ¼ cup, chopped

Cheese: 1 slice of your favorite cheese or ¼ cup of your favorite shredded cheese, or 2 tablespoons cream cheese

Nuts: 1 ounce almonds, pecans, pistachios, pine nuts, macadamia nuts, Brazil nuts, walnuts, or similar

Seeds: 1 tablespoon chia seeds, flax seeds, hemp seeds, or sesame seeds

Oils: 1 tablespoon healthy oil for sautéing

Dairy: 1–2 tablespoons heavy cream, butter, or ghee

Nondairy: 1–2 tablespoons coconut milk or coconut cream

Nut/seed butters: 1 tablespoon nut or seed butter such as peanut butter, almond butter, cashew butter, macadamia butter, or sesame butter

Mayonnaise: 1 tablespoon avocado oil mayonnaise or regular mayonnaise

Dressings & Sauces: 1–2 tablespoons of any high-fat, low-carbohydrate, and low-sugar dressing or sauce

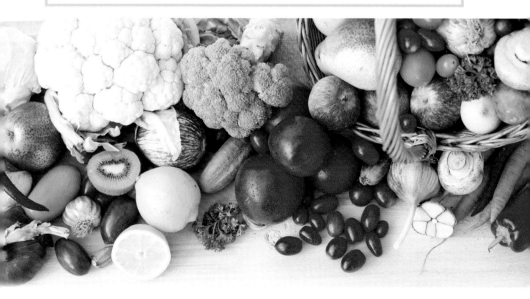

Example Breakfast Meals Using the Low-Carb Select Guidelines

Low-Carb Select Formula:
Steak (protein) +
Egg (protein) +
Cooking oil (fat) +
Asparagus (low-glycemic produce) +
Tomato (low-glycemic produce)

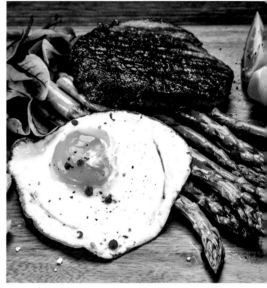

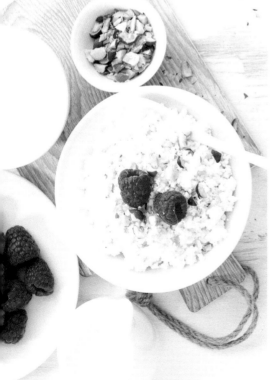

Low-Carb Select Formula:
Cottage cheese (protein) +
Nuts (fat) +
Raspberries (low-glycemic produce)

Low-Carb Select Formula:

Eggs (protein) +
Salmon (protein) +
Crème fraîche (fat) +
Diced onions (low-glycemic
  produce) +
Leafy greens (low-glycemic
  produce)

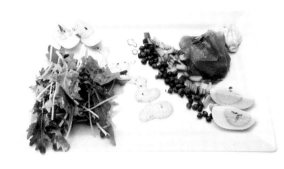

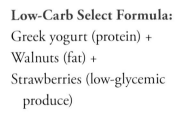

Low-Carb Select Formula:

Mushroom Omelet:
Eggs (protein) +
Cheese (fat) +
Mushrooms (low-glycemic produce) +
Sour cream (fat) +
Tomato (low-glycemic produce)

Low-Carb Select Formula:

Greek yogurt (protein) +
Walnuts (fat) +
Strawberries (low-glycemic
  produce)

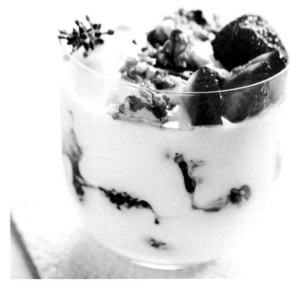

How to Meal Plan—Lunch and Dinner

Select one or two proteins (no more than 8 ounces of combined total protein between the two options for each meal), one or two fats, and one or two servings of low-glycemic produce.

Protein

Ground Beef: 6–8 ounces

Chicken or Turkey with Skin on: 6–8 ounces

Salami: 2–4 ounces

Ham: 2–4 ounces

Pork Sausage: 2–4 ounces

Eggs: 2–3 whole eggs, prepared any style

Cheese: 1–2 ounces

New York, Rib Eye, T-Bone, Sirloin, or Skirt Steak: 6–8 ounces

Filet Mignon: 6–8 ounces

Bone-in or Boneless Pork Chops: 6–8 ounces

Lamb Chops or Steaks: 6–8 ounces

Boneless, Skinless Chicken or Turkey: 6–8 ounces

Deli Turkey: 2–4 ounces

Turkey Sausage: 2–4 ounces

Ground Turkey or Chicken: 6–8 ounces

Canned Chicken or Tuna: 4–8 ounces

Fresh or Canned Salmon: 6–8 ounces

Smoked Salmon: 2–4 ounces

Trout, Mackerel, or Catfish: 6–8 ounces

Sardines, Shrimp, or Prawns: 4–8 ounces

Crab, Clams, or Mussels: 4–6 ounces

Snapper, Cod, Haddock, Sole, Halibut, or Swordfish: 6–8 ounces

Fat

Avocado: ½, sliced or mashed

Olives: ¼ cup, chopped

Cheese: 1 slice of your favorite cheese, ¼ cup of your favorite shredded cheese, or 2 tablespoons cream cheese

Nuts: 1 ounce almonds, pecans, pistachios, pine nuts, macadamia nuts, Brazil nuts, walnuts, or similar

Seeds: 1 tablespoon chia seeds, flax seeds, hemp seeds, or sesame seeds

Oils: 1 tablespoon healthy oil for sautéing

Dairy: 1 tablespoon heavy cream, butter, or ghee

Nondairy: 1–2 tablespoons coconut milk or cream

Nut/seed Butters: 1 tablespoon nut or seed butter such as peanut butter, almond butter, cashew butter, macadamia butter, or sesame butter

Bacon: 1–2 strips

Mayonnaise: 1 tablespoon avocado oil mayonnaise or regular mayonnaise

Dressings & Sauces: 1–2 tablespoons of any high-fat, low-carbohydrate, and low-sugar dressing or sauce

Low-Glycemic Produce

Zucchini: 1 cup, cooked

Spaghetti Squash: 1 cup, cooked

Fennel: ½–1 cup, cooked

Tomato: ½ cup, sliced

Avocado: ½, sliced or mashed

Bell pepper: ½ cup, sliced or diced

Mushrooms: ½ cup, sliced or diced

Onions: ¼ cup, sliced or diced

Hot peppers: ½ cup, sliced

Pickles: ½ cup, sliced

Spinach: 1 cup raw or ½ cup cooked

Kale: 1 cup raw or ½ cup cooked

Asparagus: 3–4 spears

Green Beans: 1 cup, cooked

Broccoli: ½–1 cup, cooked

Brussels Sprouts: ½–1 cup, cooked

Cucumber: ½–1 cup, sliced

Leafy Greens: 1–2 cups

Cabbage: 1–2 cups

Burger Topper Combo: 2–3 lettuce leaves, 1 large slice tomato, 1 thin slice onion

Small Mixed Salad: 1–2 cups leafy greens, ⅓ cup diced tomato/onion, 1 half avocado, sliced

Sandwich Lettuce Cup Combo: 2–4 large lettuce leaf cups, ⅓ cup diced tomato/onion, 1 half avocado, sliced

Mixed Produce: 1–2 cups any mixed low-glycemic produce

Example Lunch and Dinner Meals Using the Low-Carb Select Guidelines

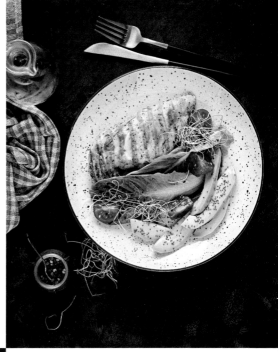

Low-Carb Select Formula:

Chicken (protein) +

Cooking oil (fat) +

Avocado (fat) +

Leafy greens (low-glycemic produce) +

Tomato (low-glycemic produce)

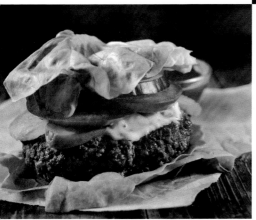

Low-Carb Select Formula:

Ground beef (protein) +

Mayonnaise (fat) +

Burger topper combo (low-glycemic produce) +

Pickles (low-glycemic produce)

Low-Carb Select Formula:
Eggs (protein) +
Mayonnaise (fat) +
Leafy greens (low-glycemic
produce)

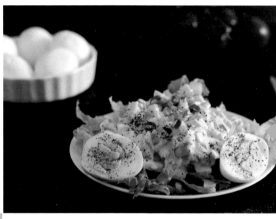

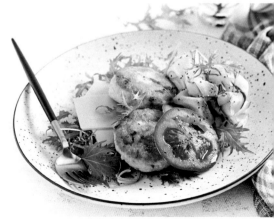

Low-Carb Select Formula:
Shrimp (protein) +
Avocado (fat) +
Pesto (fat) +
Parmesan cheese (fat) +
Spinach (low-glycemic produce) +
Zucchini noodles (low-glycemic
produce)

Low-Carb Select Formula:
Ground chicken (protein) +
Cooking oil (fat) +
Cheese (fat) +
Cucumber (low-glycemic
produce) +
Burger topper combo (low-
glycemic produce)

Low-Carb Select Formula:

Salmon (protein) +

Feta cheese (fat) +

Olives (fat) +

Mixed produce (low-
   glycemic produce)

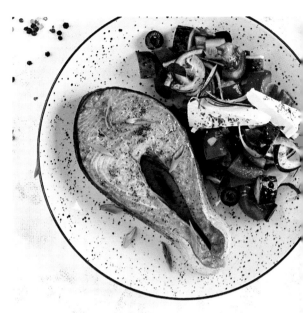

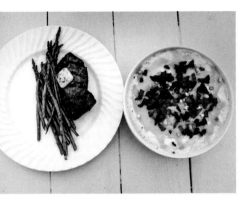

Low-Carb Select Formula:

Steak (protein) +

Loaded cauliflower: Cauliflower
   (low-glycemic produce) +

Cheese (fat) +

Bacon (fat) +

Asparagus (low-glycemic produce)

✳   ✳   ✳

As a reminder, not all low-carb-approved foods are found in this chapter—please refer to chapter 5 if you're looking for additions or substitutions. The Low-Carb Select Meal Planning System employs common, easy-to-find foods that most mainstream grocery stores carry. For a variety of unique breakfast, lunch, dinner, side dish, sauce, and dressing recipes, refer to chapters 19, 20, 21, and 22.

CHAPTER 14
All of Your Questions, Answered

If you have questions about what you have read so far, you will probably find the answers in this chapter. Essentially, you can consider the answers to these questions as rules to follow while following the low-carb protocol. Some of the "rules" may seem strict at first but your body will adjust, you will see incredible results, and your relationship with food will make a drastic change. Those who adopt this lifestyle realize they may have previously been consuming excessive amounts of sugar, carbohydrates, and processed foods. Improvements in how you feel and the noticeable changes in your body will convince you to not resort back to the standard American diet of excessive amounts of sugar, breads, pastas, cereals, crackers, and processed foods. These rules are in place to help take the guesswork out of your eating plan, and you will also find solutions to common roadblocks.

Q1 What are medical-grade weight loss products? Should I use them, and where do I find them?

Medical-grade weight loss products are specially formulated, prepackaged, low-carbohydrate and high-protein foods that look and taste like your old favorites. They include (but are not limited to) pasta, cereal, crackers, chips, bars, candies, shakes, drinks, and entrées. The preparation phase found in chapter 6 offers a questionnaire in order to evaluate whether or not medical-grade weight loss products may be a good fit for you. If you decide to implement them into your low-carbohydrate nutrition plan, you can order your products at doctorsweightloss.com.

(Q2) If I decide to use medical-grade weight loss products, how does that work?

The most popular regimen is called the Accelerated Plan and that consists of three to four medical-grade weight loss products per day and one sensible meal. Your sensible meal will consist of protein, vegetables, an optional low-sugar fruit, and an optional healthy fat. The Lifestyle Plan consists of two to three products and two sensible meals per day, and the Maintenance Plan consists of one to two products and three sensible meals per day. You can read more about each of these plans on pages 55, 63, and 68.

(Q3) What do I do if I don't want to use medical-grade weight loss products?

You can follow the low-carb grocery lists and meal plans found in chapters 5, 10, 11, 12, 13, and 15. You will learn everything you need to know to formulate a quick and easy high-protein, low-carb, and low-sugar nutrition plan.

(Q4) How much is the average weight loss per month for the plan which incorporates medical-grade weight loss products versus the plan that doesn't incorporate products?

If followed accurately, the average weight loss per month for the product plans is fifteen pounds, however, many lose as much as twenty to twenty-five pounds per month. If followed accurately, the average weight loss per month for the non-product plans is ten pounds; however, some lose as much as fifteen to twenty pounds per month.

Q5 I have done similar plans with medical-grade weight loss products in the past and there were "limited" and "unlimited" products, meaning some were higher in carbs and sugars so I couldn't consume more than one of those per day. Are Doctors Weight Loss products limited and unlimited?

Yes! You are only allowed one "limited" product per day, and the rest should be "unlimited," however, if you end up consuming two limited products on some days, you'll still get results as your overall carbohydrate and sugar consumption will still be far lower than the typical diet. The unlimited products have no more than 9 grams of carbs and 5 grams of sugar per serving. The limited products have more than 9 grams of carbs and 5 grams of sugar per serving.

Q6 If I decide to do a medical-grade weight loss plan, how long should I stay on it? And what do I do once I'd like to get off the product plan?

The Doctors Weight Loss product plans are safe to stay on for several months so you should try to adhere to your plan until you have reached within five pounds of your goal weight. You can either wean off the products slowly with the lifestyle and maintenance plans found in chapters 8 and 9, or you can skip straight to a low-carb meal plan which consists of only grocery fare, found in chapters 10, 11, and 13.

Q7 Do I need to take vitamins and minerals if I'm on a product plan?

No, you do not. Many of the Doctors Weight Loss products are fortified with nutrients, and you will also get a plethora of vitamins and minerals from the required and optional servings of vegetables, leafy greens, low-sugar fruits, and healthy fats.

Q8 In a quick summary, what can and can't I eat on my low-carb plan?

You *can* eat low-carbohydrate vegetables, extremely low-sugar fruits, seafood, meat, poultry, eggs, cheese, cottage cheese, plain yogurt, cream, butter, nuts, seeds, oils, dark chocolate, and low-carb condiments such as mayonnaise, dressings, and sauces. You *cannot* consume bread, cereal, pasta, rice, crackers, potatoes (unless they are medical-grade weight loss products), moderate- or high-carbohydrate fruits and vegetables, starches, sugary foods, soda, fruit juice, or typical dessert foods.

Q9 What are macronutrients and why are they important to know about?

Fats, carbohydrates, and proteins are the three macronutrients found in the diet. For the Doctors Weight Loss regimen, carbohydrate intake should be between 10 and 20 percent, protein intake should be between 50 and 60 percent, and fat should be between 20 and 40 percent. Macronutrients should not be confused with micronutrients, which consist of vitamins and minerals.

Q10 How many grams of carbohydrates should I have per day?

This is a tricky question since we are all different, so carbohydrate needs will vary from person to person. Generally speaking, you should consume no more than 95 grams of carbohydrates per day, but it is certainly beneficial to stick to 50 grams of total carbohydrates or less per day, or 25 grams of net carbohydrates (total carbohydrates minus grams of fiber) or less per day, if you feel comfortable doing so. You will still get results if you feel that 95 grams of carbs per day is more your speed, but they may not happen quite as quickly.

Q11 How do I track all of my carbohydrates, fats, and proteins?

Contact us by emailing info@doctorsweightloss.com to get your complimentary food tracking system which includes thousands of standard groceries, as well as the Doctors Weight Loss medical-grade weight loss products. If you're worried about this being too much work, it will only last two to three weeks before you become accustomed to knowing what foods have the proper amount of carbohydrates, fats, and proteins for your nutrition plan. Although this process may seem daunting in the beginning, it gets extremely easy and then before you know it, you won't need to track anymore as you will know what is in most foods.

Q12 Do I need to track my calories, too?

People of different heights, weights, ages, activity levels, and goals all have assorted calorie requirements. Not to mention, when it comes to weight loss, calories in versus calories expended will always matter to some degree. Even if you hit your macro requirements in perfect ranges, you could still fail to lose weight (or even gain weight) if you overeat too many calories. Your complimentary Doctors Weight Loss tracking system will help you determine how many calories you should consume to maintain or lose weight.

Q13 Will the fats found in this diet make my cholesterol worse?

One of the primary guidelines of *The Doctors Weight Loss Diet* is to choose the healthiest fats possible. Fats found in foods such as avocado, extra-virgin olive oil, nuts, seeds, and wild salmon actually help promote good cholesterol. If one focuses on unhealthy fats such as inferior oils and processed meats, then it is possible that negative outcomes such as increased bad cholesterol and excessive sodium levels could occur. There are several studies which show that a nutrition plan which includes healthy fats is associated with improvements in good cholesterol, cardio-vascular risk, and type 2 diabetes.[17]

 Will I get enough fiber and micronutrients?

If your 10 to 20 percent allotted carbohydrates are dedicated to mostly green vegetables and low-sugar fruits, you will definitely get the required fiber, vitamin, and mineral intake. The average American only consumes 10 to 15 grams of fiber per day so if you plan correctly, you can double the amount of fiber that the average person gets if you watch what you eat. The table below illustrates one example (there are several other combinations in which you can achieve this with different produce) of how you can get 24 grams of fiber while remaining under the lower limit of 25 grams of net carbohydrates. Not to mention, the consumption of this many servings of low-sugar produce will give a substantial amount of essential vitamins, minerals, and antioxidants.

Food	Net Carbohydrates	Fiber
1 cup cooked spinach	2g	4g
2 cups chopped romaine lettuce	1g	2g
2 cups cooked broccoli	12g	10g
½ cup raspberries	7g	8g
Totals	**22g**	**24g**

 Will I have to spend a lot of time cooking?

Typically speaking, some cooking and food preparation does come along with the territory of living a healthy lifestyle. If you are not using the prepackaged medical-grade weight loss products, you will need to spend an average of three hours per week (or twenty-five minutes per day) in the kitchen to execute your plan. Of course, it could be done in less time if you eat in restaurants frequently (refer to chapter 15 for your

---

17 Kosinski, Christophe, and François R Jornayvaz. "Effects of Ketogenic Diets on Cardiovascular Risk Factors: Evidence from Animal and Human Studies." Nutrients. MDPI, May 19, 2017. https://www.ncbi.nlm.nih.gov/pmc/articles/PMC5452247/.

guides to low-carb restaurant and fast-food fare), or if you are already used to meal-prepping. If you decide to implement the Doctors Weight Loss Accelerated Plan (three to four medical-grade weight loss products per day and one sensible meal), your average weekly cooking time will be around one hour.

(Q16) So, I can eat in restaurants? Can I do that often?

Yes, you can! Some who are looking to lose weight or improve health are reluctant to even try a low-carb nutrition plan as they assume restaurants will be off limits. Let's face it, a large percentage of the population eat in restaurants on a regular basis due to work obligations, social gatherings, and just for convenience. We have dedicated chapter 15 to those who fall into this category. You will find several examples of typical restaurant scenarios and how to modify your meal to make them low in carbohydrates.

(Q17) Can I get fast food too?

We are looking to optimize health and wellness (in addition to achieving weight loss) so while you can eat in restaurants fairly often, we will suggest minimizing fast food intake. Reason being is fast food consists of inferior ingredients and detrimental additives. Of course, if you're in a pinch and fast food is the only option, refer to chapter 15 for a list of the most popular fast food chains and how to order low-carb meals at each of them.

(Q18) I always eat things like sandwiches and cereal—what will I replace those items with?

There are many common mainstream foods that are a part of the standard American diet, but they are not allowed on the low-carb nutrition plan due to higher carbohydrate and sugar content. This table of simple low-carb food swaps will help you navigate the best and tastiest substitutions. Keep in mind, if you opt for a product plan, you will still get to eat specially formulated low-carb pasta, cereal, chips, and desserts!

Instead of This	Have This
Cheeseburger on a bun	Cheeseburger with no bun, or wrapped in lettuce
Sandwich on bread	Sandwich fillings wrapped in lettuce or over a bed of greens
Chicken pasta dish	Chicken with riced cauliflower or zucchini noodles and sauce
Steak with potatoes	Steak with vegetables or salad
Sugary salad with cranberries, candied nuts, and sweet dressing	Salad with nuts, cheese, avocado, protein, and savory oil-based dressing
Sides like French fries, rice, potato, bread, or pasta	Extra vegetables topped with butter or oil, mashed or riced cauliflower, small side salad topped with oil-based dressing
Chicken fingers or other breaded proteins with ketchup	Grilled chicken or other grilled proteins with creamy dipping sauce such as avocado oil mayonnaise
Tacos in tortillas	Lettuce-wrapped tacos
Burritos in tortillas	Burrito bowls with protein, vegetables, cheese, avocado, sour cream, and salsa
Piece of toast with peanut butter	Celery sticks with peanut butter
Ice cream	Berries topped with heavy whipping cream
Bread basket	Charcuterie board with cheese, meats, olives, and nuts
Dessert of cookies or baked goods	Red wine with dark chocolate and cheese
Standard breakfast with omelet, bacon, potatoes, and toast	Omelet with cheese, bacon, and sliced tomatoes or berries
Sweetened coffee beverage	Unsweetened coffee with coconut oil, cream, butter, or MCT oil
Salted chips	Salted nuts

(Q19) Can I eat any sort of fat to fulfill my 20 to 40 percent fat guideline?

We urge against a "free-for-all" of consuming any and all fats just for the sake of fulfilling your macronutrient quotas. Most people do not consume enough omega-3 fatty acids because only certain foods contain them. Omega-3 fats are not produced by our bodies, so we need to get them from our diet; they assist with brain function, heart health, and reducing inflammation. Good fats also help our blood sugar levels remain even and they can help us feel full for longer. Some examples of foods that have the healthiest fats are oysters, egg yolks, salmon, mackerel, grass-fed beef, avocado oil, olive oil, walnuts, macadamia nuts, chia seeds, and avocado.

(Q20) Do I have to pack my food?

Packing a healthy lunch or at least some healthy snacks to have around the office or at school is one of the most efficient ways to combat workplace donuts and vending machines because if you're not hungry, passing up the treats is far easier. We don't want you spending hours in your kitchen, so if you're unsure of how to quickly prepare lunches, simply double up on your dinner recipe and pack half of it to go, or grab a low-carb-approved meal at a restaurant or café (see chapter 15 for those guidelines).

(Q21) If I cave and eat something sugary or with lots of carbohydrates, do I have to quit and start over?

No! Jump back on that wagon immediately! Many popular diets require one to start over if a piece (or even a bite) of cake at a birthday party occurs. This train of thought can lead to reluctance, and even anxiety when it comes to taking the first step to making a lifestyle change. There is misconception that proper nutrition has to be followed 100 percent of the time, and there is no wiggle room if you want to see results, but that can't be further from the truth. You will see progress (and lots of it) if you adhere to the Doctors Weight Loss principles and strategies most of the time. There may be situations when a slip-up occurs—acknowledge it, don't feel guilty about it, and jump right back on the wagon.

 Can I ever eat a high-carb food?

The short answer is yes, but this really depends on individual preferences. In theory, if you were extremely low in carbohydrates all day and then wanted one serving of a food that was higher in carbohydrates, you could still fall into your daily guideline of carbohydrates.

The low-carb diet can seem daunting and hard to understand—we hope this "Q and A" chapter has cleared up any confusion. Like any nutrition lifestyle, once you sort out the facts and get into a routine, you'll find that it is pretty simple. Once you complete your first thirty days of the Doctors Weight Loss protocol, you'll be so well-versed that the days of tracking macronutrients or searching for questions and answers will be over!

CHAPTER 15
How to Follow Your Program While Dining Out

If you have absolutely no time for food prepping, or you just have zero interest or motivation to pack food for work, you can certainly eat in restaurants, order takeout, or even have the occasional fast food. In today's society, it's commonplace to grab food (even every day!) during your lunch hour in a restaurant or at a takeout establishment. This is reality for many of us, so we want to provide a strategy for low-carb weight loss even if you're a frequent restaurant-goer. Let's face it, life happens (and so do work luncheons, birthdays, and other social gatherings), and we want you to have options so you can live your life accordingly. Many think they have to give up their social lives or drastically rearrange their eating schedule at the office to adhere to the low-carb lifestyle, and that can lead to procrastination for even starting a nutrition plan due to strict limitations. Yes, you can still go to restaurants and enjoy wonderful company (and maybe even a glass of wine . . . or two).

Fast food is permitted, but we advise to limit it to the odd occasion because we want you to achieve wellness in addition to weight loss. We have heard countless stories of low-carb dieters sticking to the proper macronutrients of fats, carbohydrates, and proteins by frequenting the fast-food drive-through and ordering a bunless double (or triple) cheeseburger with mayonnaise, along with a diet soda, which is definitely not ideal. It's an easy habit to get into since it's convenient, relatively cheap, and pretty tasty! Especially if you're new to the low-carb life and learning the ropes, we want to set the healthiest foundation possible and instruct readers how to get the best nutrition from this type of food plan since choosing detrimental foods (even while hitting your macronutrient requirements) can lead to unfavorable outcomes. If you're in a true bind, then having one fast-food meal per week, maximum, should not sabotage your health and wellness goals.

Dining establishments that can be frequented often include:
- National chain dine-in restaurants.
- Smaller boutique dine-in restaurants.
- Take-out restaurants that offer salads, sandwiches (lettuce-wrapped), and platters with choices of unprocessed meats and vegetables.
- Coffee shops.

You'll want to limit regular use of:
- Standard fast-food establishments.
- Almost anything with a drive-through.
- Pizza parlors.
- Takeout places that only offer processed deli meats.

It's convenient to look online at restaurant menus before choosing where to grab your meal as some have far more low-carb-approved options than others. If you end up somewhere without looking at food options first, not to worry—you can get a suitable meal almost anywhere nowadays! Of course, you may have to modify your order, but making simple sub-stitutions will turn a high-glycemic meal into a low-carb-friendly one quite easily. Below are ten common restaurant scenarios which include high-carbohydrate and high-sugar foods, as well as low-carb replacement options.

Scenario One:
You're at a typical cafe and the server arrives with a basket of bread and butter.

Solution 1: Before the bread even touches the table, just say "no thanks!"—you'll be eating a full meal soon anyway.

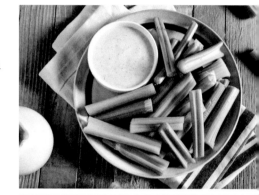

Solution 2: Replace with veggies and a low-carb dip.

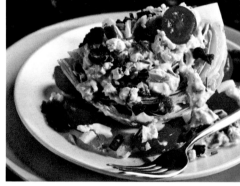

Solution 3: Replace with a small starter salad with a cream-based dressing.

Solution 4: Replace with a low-carbohydrate, cheese- or cream-based soup.

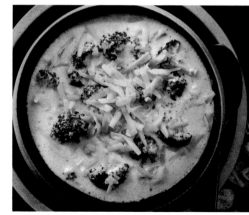

Scenario Two:
You're at a more casual takeout place with sandwiches, salads, and burgers.

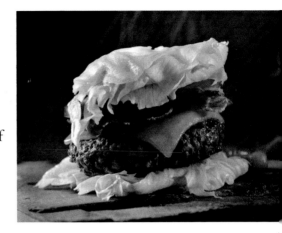

Solution 1: Just get it lettuce-wrapped—most restaurants will oblige. Sorry, no fries, but a side of green vegetables will do!

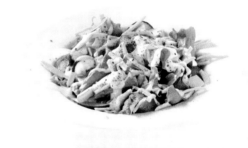

Solution 2: Not only will most takeout establishments lettuce-wrap burgers, you can get sandwiches lettuce-wrapped too, or you can even ask for a "sub in a tub" to have all of your favorite sandwich fillings in a bowl.

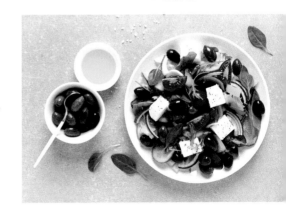

Solution 3: A hearty salad with fats that will keep you satiated—choose a dressing that is typically low in sugar such as oil and vinegar.

Scenario Three:
You're at an Italian eatery and everyone is getting pasta.

Solution 1: Beef carpaccio with additions such as arugula, cheese, olives, and tomatoes.

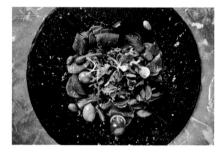

Solution 2: Any typical Italian protein dish such as chicken, meat, or fish, but with no added pasta.

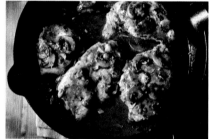

Solution 3: Caprese salad topped with olive oil.

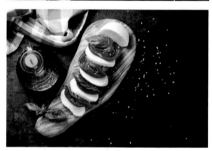

Solution 4: Not all, but many Italian restaurants now offer zoodles (zucchini noodles) with meat sauce or meatballs. If this option isn't available, ask for meat sauce or meatballs with a side of green veggies or squash.

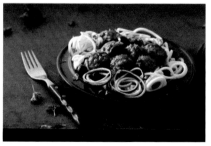

---

*   Sorry, but no cauliflower crust pizza in restaurants is allowed—they are typically made with a mixture of wheat flour and cauliflower flour.

Scenario Four:
You're at a typical chain restaurant with standard meals that contain a protein with side dishes of pasta, rice, and potatoes.

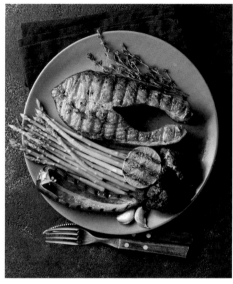

Solution 1: Ask your server to remove all high-carbohydrate side dishes and replace with low-carbohydrate produce.

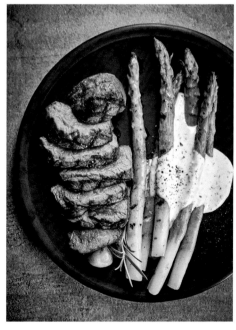

Solution 2: Ask your server to remove all high-carbohydrate sides dishes and ask to replace with one green vegetable with a cheese-, cream-, or butter-based sauce.

Scenario Five:
You're at happy hour with friends for drinks and small plates.

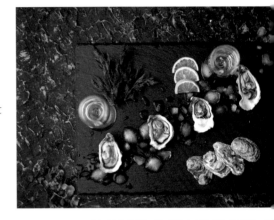

Solution 1: You celebrate your new low-carb lifestyle with brut sparkling wine and oysters.

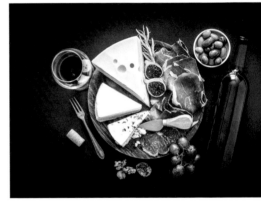

Solution 2: You relax with a glass of cabernet sauvignon and a cheese board with nuts and olives.

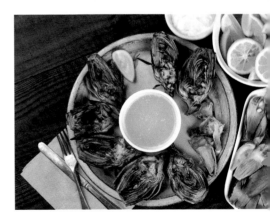

Solution 3: You pair a buttery chardonnay with a steamed artichoke with mayonnaise and butter for dipping.

Scenario Six:
You're grabbing Mexican food for taco Tuesday.

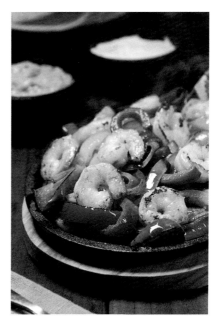

Solution 1: Shrimp, steak, or chicken fajitas with guacamole, shredded cheese, and salsa— ask for lettuce cups or eat as a platter.

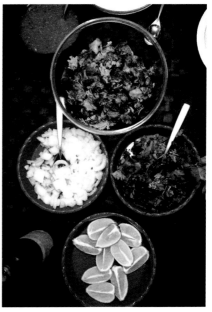

Solution 2: Chile verde platter of pork, green sauce, sour cream, and guacamole—skip the rice, beans, and tortillas!

Scenario Seven:
You're out for Chinese or Vietnamese food, or for sushi.

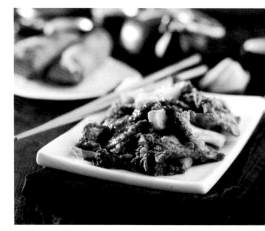

Solution 1: Beef and broccoli and egg drop soup instead of a noodle dish.

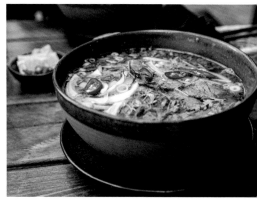

Solution 2: Vietnamese pho—ask for no noodles and extra veggies and herbs, which is a standard option on most menus!

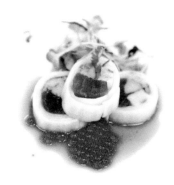

Solution 3: At sushi, instead of a roll with rice, ask for it to be wrapped in cucumber—this, too, is a standard option on most menus!

Scenario Eight:
You pop into Starbucks before work.

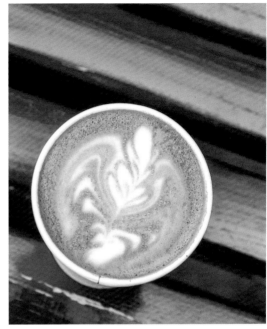

Solution 1: A grande coffee with heavy cream or almond milk, or a grande latte made with heavy cream instead of milk.

Solution 2: Egg bites (eggs with cheese and veggies, or with cheese and bacon), string cheese, and mashed avocado. These items are offered à la carte and make an easy low-carb-approved breakfast on the go.

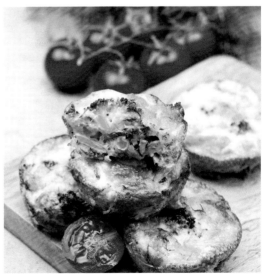

Scenario Nine:
You're out to breakfast or brunch with family and friends.

Solution 1: Omelet with vegetables, cheese, and sausage with small side of tomatoes and/or berries, and coffee.

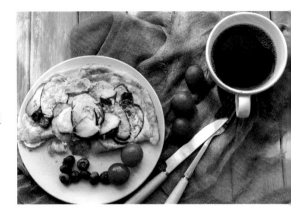

Solution 2: Eggs Benedict with no bread base (most restaurants will make it this way); ask to add fresh produce such as asparagus, tomatoes, and mushrooms.

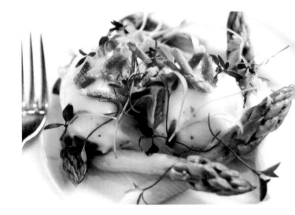

Scenario Ten:
You're at a sports bar watching Sunday football.

Solution 1: Wings, celery, and blue cheese.

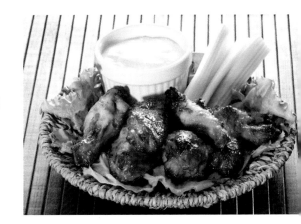

Solution 2: Baby back ribs (no sugary glaze) with green vegetables or a side salad.

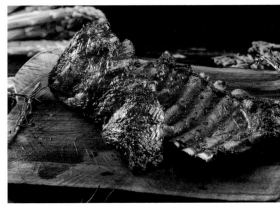

Solution 3: Cobb salad with chicken or turkey, bacon, hard-boiled egg, tomatoes, avocado, and cheese.

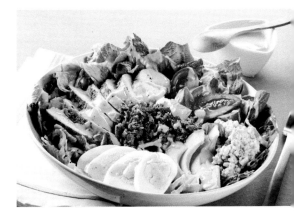

Scenario Eleven:
You're trying some Greek cuisine.

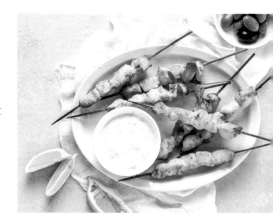

Solution 1: Chicken souvlaki (kebobs) with cucumber yogurt dipping sauce and a side of olives.

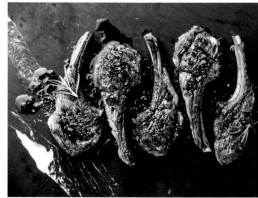

Solution 2: Lamb chops with haricots verts or green beans.

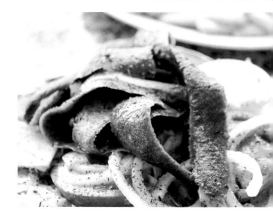

Solution 3: Gyro platter—skip the pita!

Scenario Twelve:
You're at a fine-dining establishment to celebrate a special occasion.

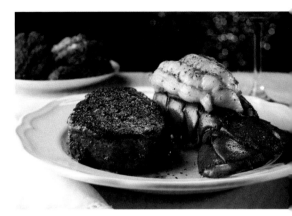

Solution 1: Steak and lobster with a green vegetable and a glass of red wine.

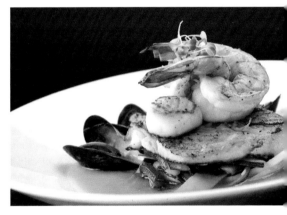

Solution 2: An eclectic seafood dish with fish, shellfish, and low-glycemic produce.

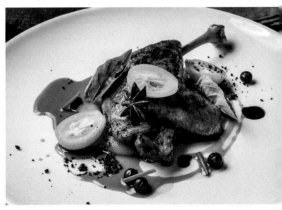

Solution 3: A fancy poultry dish such as duck confit with low-sugar fruits and greens.

Scenario Thirteen:
You pick a traditional steak house for some dinner.

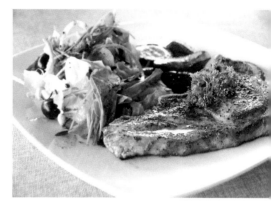

Solution 1: A juicy pork chop with vegetables and a side salad.

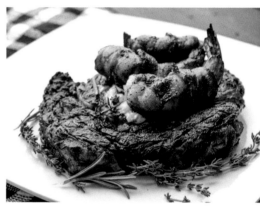

Solution 2: A rib eye with bacon-wrapped shrimp.

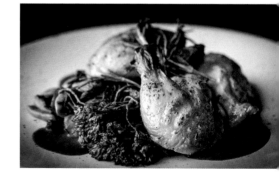

Solution 3: Roasted chicken with broccolini and mushrooms.

Low-Carb Fast-Food Options

It doesn't get any simpler than grabbing some fast food while still sticking to your low-carb nutrition plan. Of course, we recommend limiting fast food, but if you're in a bind, it can be super simple to swing by a drive-through. We want to give you the best options if you find yourself in this situation, but try not to take advantage of these low-carb fast food options more than once or twice per week as true health (not just weight loss) is our top priority for you. Just to have in your back pocket for emergencies, below you will find some of the most popular American fast food dining establishments, along with how to order low-carb-friendly meals at each one.

McDonald's

McDonald's has adjusted to the low-carb needs of many dieters. Essentially, you can order any burger or breakfast sandwich and simply say "no bun and no ketchup," and they will package your burger on a plate or bowl with meat, cheese, lettuce, a sprinkling of onions, and a slice or two of pickles. You can ask for mayonnaise, ranch, and/or mustard on the side—sorry, but mainstream ketchup is a bit too high in sugar! The breakfast sandwiches will be served in the same way with egg, cheese, and sausage on a plate. Keep in mind, you can use this McDonald's order strategy at most other burger-based fast-food chains as they, too, are privy to the needs of low-carb dieters. There are at least twenty items to choose from at McDonald's, but some of the most popular ones can be ordered as follows:

- Any cheeseburger (single, double, triple) with no bun and no ketchup.
- Any breakfast sandwich with no muffin.
- Bacon Ranch Grilled Chiken Salad with no tomatoes and no dressing (sub ranch dipping sauce).
- Artisan grilled chicken sandwich with no bun. Sorry, but the nuggets and crispy chicken sandwich are off-limits due to being encased in breading.

Subway

The term "sub in a tub" was coined at Jersey Mike's, however, this is also used at other fast-food sandwich establishments. You can get your favorite sandwich fillings in a "tub" or bowl, with the bread. In addition to the sandwich bowls, Subway offers a variety of salads and breakfast items. Here's how to order some of their most popular low-carb items:

- 6-inch bacon, egg, and cheese sub with no bread.
- 6-inch tuna sub plain with no bread.
- 6-inch cold cut combo sub plain with no bread.
- 6-inch oven-roasted chicken plain with no bread.
- Black forest ham salad.
- Chicken and bacon ranch salad.
- Spicy Italian salad.

Burger King

As with McDonald's, you can ask for any burger or breakfast sandwich with no bun and no sauce and it will be served on a platter or in a bowl. There are some other unique low-carb orders at Burger King below:

- Eggnormous burrito in a bowl with no tortilla or hash browns; add a black coffee with cream on the side.
- You can replace French fry sides with a side salad but remember to ask for no croutons.
- You can add ranch or Buffalo dipping sauce to any order.

Taco Bell

Just as you would order a burger with no bun, you can order tacos and burritos with no tortillas and Taco Bell will know what to do—you'll get a bowl or platter. To take it up even one more notch, there are low-carb-friendly power bowls that are loaded with additional ingredients such as guacamole and sour cream. Here are some of the most popular low-carb finds at Taco Bell:

- Steak or Chicken Burrito Supreme with no tortilla and no beans. You will get a bowl of protein, lettuce, diced tomatoes, diced onions, and a little bit of low-carbohydrate sauce.
- Chicken quesadilla melt with no tortilla. You will get a platter of melty cheese, chicken, and a little sauce to enjoy with a fork.
- The Grilled Chicken Power Bowl is packed with chicken, lettuce, guacamole, avocado ranch dressing, sour cream, and pico de gallo. Make sure to ask for no rice and beans, and feel free to add some hot sauce.

Wendy's

As with other popular fast-food chains, Wendy's is known for its burgers but they also have other selections to choose from. Aside from the typical lettuce-wrapped burger order, here are some popular menu items. You can add the Caesar salad dressing, classic ranch dressing, or southwest ranch dressing to any salad or sandwich.

- Breakfast Baconator with no bun.
- Grilled chicken sandwich with no bun and no sauce.
- Southwest avocado grilled chicken salad.
- Parmesan grilled chicken Caesar salad.

Dunkin' Donuts

There is actually more to Dunkin' Donuts than just donuts, so if you're in a bind and need a quick breakfast, you can still pay them a visit (if the smell of the donuts won't derail your plan). Feel free to order any of their numerous hot and cold brews and unsweetened teas (just add cream). If you to add a syrup to your drink, flavor shots are part of the secret menu and they are sugar-free. You can order any of the following "Wake-Up Wraps" but just ask to hold the wrap.

- Sausage, egg, and cheese.
- Bacon, egg, and cheese.
- Ham, egg, and cheese.
- Turkey sausage, egg white, and cheese.
- Egg and cheese.

Chick-Fil-A

Just like ordering a burger with no bun, you'll do the same with the chicken sandwiches and breakfast sandwiches at Chick-Fil-A. There are some other notable items (besides the sandwiches) that are low-carb-friendly, and here's how to order them:

- Hash brown scramble bowl with no hash browns and either grilled chicken or sausage.
- Grilled chicken nuggets with zesty Buffalo sauce or garden and herb ranch sauce.
- Cobb salad with grilled chicken, topped with light Italian dressing or avocado lime ranch dressing.

Pizza Hut

Pizza parlors may be the most difficult restaurants in which to stay low-carb, but there are some options. If temptation is not a problem, you can order any pizza with lots of toppings and eat the toppings only. Sorry, but cauliflower crusts are not allowed in a pizza establishment, because they are typically made with a percentage of cauliflower flour and a (usually) larger percentage of wheat flour. Here are a few low-carb orders at Pizza Hut, and you will, most likely, find similar items at other pizza chains:

- Caesar salad
- Chicken Caesar salad

- Any order of wings with no breading and no glaze; add blue cheese or ranch for dipping.

Panda Express

Ordering at Panda Express can be tricky as many seemingly low-carb dishes are doused in sugary sauces. After meticulously going through their nutrition menu, you will find these to be the only suitable options, and of course all noodle and rice sides will need to be omitted.

- Super greens entrée.
- Grilled teriyaki chicken.
- Grilled Asian chicken.
- Steamed ginger fish.

Sonic Drive-In

You'll use the same burger ordering techniques at Sonic since they have several burger and chicken sandwiches. There is one other unique low-carb option that you won't find at most other fast-food establishments and here's how you order it.

- All-American hot dog with no bun, no relish, and no ketchup. The hot dog will be served with mustard and diced onions and if you need more than one, you'll still fall in line with your macros.

Chipotle Mexican Grill

Chipotle has really jumped on the low-carb wagon for their customers by adding a section of the menu called "Lifestyle Bowls." Here you will find several meals that are labeled as "keto," "paleo," and "Whole30," which have ingredients such as protein, cauliflower rice, avocado, and cheese, so you don't have to alter your order to make it low-carb. Here are the most popular low-carb meals, and you can order them as is—simple as that!

- Keto salad bowl (served with greens, chicken, salsa, Jack cheese, and avocado).
- Keto bowl (served with cilantro-lime cauliflower rice, chicken, salsa, Jack cheese, and avocado).

Even if your favorite fast-food establishment was not found in this chapter, the techniques for ordering will remain the same for most other chains. Just remember the general rules of thumb—skip the buns, bread, tortillas, and fries, and beware of any high-sugar sauces. As a reminder, while you can still hit your low-carb macros with fast food, we suggest limiting these types of meals for when you're in a pinch for time so you achieve overall health and wellness, in addition to weight loss.

Contrary to popular belief, the low-carb nutrition plan can be achieved even if you frequent dining establishments—you just have to be a little meticulous about your order! As with anything, once you establish a routine, ordering the most effective meals at any type of restaurant will become second nature. Of course, it's always best to prepare your own meals so you can choose the healthiest ingredients, but if that's just not realistic for your lifestyle, you can still get the weight loss results by following the simple guidelines found in this chapter.

CHAPTER 16

How to Manage or Prevent Type 2 Diabetes with Food

Type 2 diabetes affects millions of men and women every year. Research shows that this condition may be prevented and/or treated through good nutrition and exercise. Since prediabetes and type 2 diabetes is on the rise, it is imperative to take precautions by implementing a low-sugar nutrition plan that is adopted as a lifestyle, as opposed to a short-term diet. If you are reading this chapter because you have been diagnosed with type 2 diabetes, we have specialized nutrition guidelines for you! Please keep in mind, if you have been diagnosed with type 2 diabetes, please follow your doctor's orders and get immediate attention, as it can be very dangerous if not treated.

You may be wondering what to eat to prevent type 2 diabetes from occurring in the first place. All of the nutrition information outlined in this book will help to lower your risk of developing the condition. Avoiding sugar, as well as consuming the proper amounts and types of carbohydrates, is imperative to efficiently manage blood sugar levels. Not all carbohydrates demonstrate the same qualities and the effects they have on the human body, so it is imperative to select the best carbohydrates possible. Below are some questions to ask yourself to help you identify which carbohydrate-containing foods are most beneficial for weight and blood sugar management.

Does the ingredient label contain wheat, grains, and/or gluten?
If the answer is yes, it is best to avoid this carbohydrate-containing food. Most products that contain wheat, grains, and/or gluten tend to have a high amount of carbohydrates per serving, and these types of carbs are high-glycemic, converting to a lot of sugar upon digestion. Common examples to look out for on the nutrition label are wheat, rice, corn, and oats.

Does the ingredient label on the food exhibit a long list?
If the answer is yes, it is best to avoid this carbohydrate-containing food. A long ingredient list is a strong indicator that the food is manufactured to a point of being far from a natural state, containing several toxic ingredients.

Does the food have a shelf life?
If the answer is yes, it is best to avoid this carbohydrate-containing food. Foods that have a shelf life (such as pasta, bread, crackers, chips, cookies, and cereal) tend to contain a variety of preservatives in order to create that long shelf life.

Is the food highly processed?
If the answer is yes, it is best to avoid this carbohydrate-containing food. Processed foods (which are also likely to have long shelf lives) also tend to have long ingredient lists—most of which we can't even pronounce, because they are not real foods that occur in nature. Not only do these foods have detrimental additives and preservatives, they also boast inferior fortified nutrients that have been added in the factory and do not absorb well.

Does the food have added sugar?
If the answer is yes, it is best to avoid this carbohydrate-containing food. Carbohydrates automatically turn into sugar when digested, so it is important not to add to that sugar that will naturally convert in your bloodstream.

Keep in mind that there are over 60 different names for sugar that have been found on food labels; some of the most common ones are barley malt, dextrose, rice syrup, sucrose, and high-fructose corn syrup.

The carbohydrate-containing foods that are low-carb-approved do not fall into any of the above-mentioned categories. They are nutrient-dense whole foods that are unprocessed with little to no shelf lives and have no added sugars. Below is a snapshot of some of our favorite carbohydrate foods, based on micronutrient composition and the effect they have on blood sugar levels. The carbohydrate foods to consume freely (while staying within the general guidelines of your low-carb macronutrient recommendations) are **highlighted in green**. Also included are carbohydrate foods that we recommend eliminating from your nutrition plan (**highlighted in red**).

Carbohydrate Foods to Consume	Carbohydrate Foods to Eliminate
Avocado	White bread
Kale	Whole wheat bread
Artichoke	White pasta
Broccoli	Whole wheat pasta
Collard greens	Cereal
Brussels sprouts	White crackers
Asparagus	Multigrain/Whole wheat crackers
Zucchini	Tortilla
Spinach	Pizza crust
Cauliflower	Croissants
Green beans	Muffins
Cucumber	Pita bread
Celery	White flour
Eggplant	Whole wheat flour
Tomato	Commercial granola bars
Bell pepper	Bagels
Cabbage	Sugary drinks
Blueberries	Candy
Raspberries	Cookies
Blackberries	Cake
Strawberries	Donuts
Onion	Ice cream

You may be wondering why the whole wheat versions of some items are on the list to avoid or eliminate since these counterparts are touted as items that should be consumed to avoid and/or treat type 2 diabetes. The truth of the matter is there is little difference between two pieces of white bread and two pieces of whole wheat bread with regard to their ingredients and nutritional makeup. Let's compare one leading brand of white bread to one leading brand of wheat bread below so we can see the similarities.

	White Bread	Wheat Bread
Serving Size	2 pieces (52g)	2 pieces (52g)
Calories	150	120
Fat	2g	1.5g
Carbohydrates	28g	24g
Protein	4g	6g
Sodium	180mg	220mg
Fiber	1.5g	3g
Most Abundant Ingredients per Nutrition Label	Enriched bleached flour (wheat flour, malted barley flour) water, high-fructose corn syrup	Whole wheat flour, water, high-fructose corn syrup, wheat, gluten, yeast

As you can see, there is very little difference between the white bread and the wheat bread. Traditional wisdom states that the wheat bread has double the amount of fiber and will therefore not affect blood sugar levels negatively, but that is false. That measly extra 1.5 grams of fiber when put up against the 24 grams of high-glycemic carbohydrates unfortunately will not make a substantial difference with regard to keeping your blood sugar levels even especially when combating an ingredient such as high-fructose corn syrup. It is true that fiber slows down the digestion of carbohydrates, which helps to maintain even blood sugar levels. When preventing or managing type 2 diabetes with food, we need foods that have a much higher fiber-to-carbohydrate ratio than items such as whole wheat bread. Below we compare the amounts of different foods we must eat in order to obtain 30 grams of fiber.

Food	Amount of calories you must eat to get 30 grams of fiber	Amount of carbohydrates you must eat to get 30 grams of fiber	Amount of sodium you must eat to get 30 grams of fiber
Whole Wheat Bread	1,350	270g	2025mg
Multigrain Cereal	1,275	275g	2,300mg
Whole Wheat Pasta	1,260	246g	20mg
Artichoke Hearts	200	45g	200mg
Raspberries	240	56g	4mg
Chia Seeds	385	33g	13mg

As illustrated above, the examples of whole, unprocessed foods are far superior when it comes to their fiber-to-carbohydrate ratio—these types of foods will really help to prevent or manage type 2 diabetes. In addition, they contain a variety of vitamins and minerals that are naturally occurring within the food, and therefore absorb more efficiently. You also will not have to worry about consuming undesirable, hidden ingredients such as high-fructose corn syrup. More examples of foods that have a high ratio of fiber to carbohydrates that are whole, unprocessed foods are:

Broccoli, Brussels sprouts, raspberries, blackberries, blueberries, avocado, okra, acorn squash, almonds, flax seeds, chia seeds, coconut, pumpkin seeds, cabbage, artichoke, pistachio nuts, and hemp seeds.

If you have been diagnosed with type 2 diabetes and your doctor said you can manage it with proper nutrition, we have put together the following recommendations for you. There are some cases of diabetes that do require medication so please follow your doctor's orders. If you are currently trying to combat type 2 diabetes, or you are simply taking preventative measures, the below guidelines may assist you:

(1) **Severely limit sugar:** The reality of fighting or avoiding type 2 diabetes comes down to severely limiting sugar. Consuming sugar is directly related with raising our blood sugar, which can result in or exacerbate the condition. Whether the sugar comes from a candy bar, ice cream, cookies, or even natural sources like honey or fruit, all types of sugar are problematic for diabetes.

(2) **Reduce carbohydrate intake:** Carbohydrates are broken down into sugar by the digestive system and that sugar enters the blood. In response to this, blood sugar rises and insulin is released by the pancreas, which prompts the sugar to be used as energy or to be stored in cells. Sometimes not enough insulin is created by the pancreas, and that leads to high blood sugar levels, as the sugar remains in the blood as opposed to getting used or stored. Carbohydrates affect blood sugar and insulin response more than proteins and fats, so it is imperative to reduce carbohydrate intake if you suffer from diabetes. We recommend an average of 25–95 grams of carbohydrates per day, however, this range is a general average. You may need more or less based on your height, current weight, desired weight, age, and activity level.

(3) **Obtain the majority of carbohydrates from vegetables:** It is still important to eat some carbohydrates, however, your primary carbohydrates should come from vegetable sources as they are low-glycemic. The glycemic index ranks carbohydrates in terms of how quickly they turn to sugar once digested. Most vegetables (notably green vegetables) are low-glycemic which means they raise blood sugar very minimally and slowly while providing energy, nutrients, and fiber.

(4) **Eliminate carbohydrates from high-sugar fruits:** Like vegetables, low-glycemic fruits are another carbohydrate source that provide essential nutrients and antioxidants while resulting in marginal blood sugar increase and insulin response. Fruits such as avocado, tomato, and bell pepper are extremely low in carbohydrates and sugar, so those can

be a part of your diabetes nutrition plan. Low-sugar fruits such as berries can be consumed in moderation (we recommend no more than one serving per day). High-glycemic fruits such as mango, figs, banana, and pineapple should be avoided as they cause spikes in the blood sugar and insulin response.

(5) **Eat more proteins and healthy fats:** Protein and healthy fats have very little bearing on blood sugar so consuming more of these macronutrients (and less carbohydrates) is key to treating or preventing type 2 diabetes. Protein and fats help keep your blood sugar levels even, and they assist with keeping you fuller for longer, which may prevent spikes and drops in blood glucose. High carbohydrate intake results in those spikes in blood sugar, followed by a "crash," which may lead to cravings for more carbohydrates. Keep in mind, it is critical to consume high-quality proteins and healthy fats (since not all proteins and fats are created equally). Wild salmon, organic meats/poultry, nuts, seeds, broccoli, spinach, avocado, and extra-virgin olive oil are great examples of proteins and fats to consume while items such as hot dogs, fried foods, vegetable oil, and fast foods are best to be avoided.

(6) **Do not eat any grain- or gluten-foods such as bread, pasta, crackers, and cereals (not even the whole wheat versions):** Grain- and gluten-containing foods such as bread, pasta, crackers, and cereals are high glycemic—they will raise your blood sugar very quickly, which triggers a substantial insulin response. The glycemic index ranks carbohydrate-containing foods with regard to how they are compared to sugar in terms of the rise in blood sugar they cause. Pure sugar is given a ranking of 100, meaning pure sugar will raise your blood sugar the most. Any item that receives a ranking of 70 or more is considered high glycemic and should be eliminated. The average commercial white bread is given a glycemic index score of 75, whereas the average commercial wheat bread is given a score of 74. So, yes, technically whole wheat bread is "better" than white bread, but it is only marginally better and will still cause substantial rises in blood sugar as it is right on the border of being considered "high-glycemic." For a reference point, carbohydrate sources such as broccoli, kale, cauliflower, tomato, Brussels sprouts, collard greens, and lettuces have glycemic index scores that are less than 20.

(7) **Do not eat gluten-free versions of bread, pasta, crackers, and cereals:** You may be wondering if the gluten-free versions of these foods are acceptable to consume while trying to manage or prevent type 2 diabetes, and the short answer is no. Gluten-free breads, pastas, crackers, and convenience foods are processed with replacement flours such as potato starch and tapioca starch. Unfortunately, these starches raise your blood sugar even more than typical gluten-containing wheat flours found in regular breads, pastas, and crackers. Even though these items are technically gluten-free, this label does not automatically mean they are healthy, as they will only do a disservice to one who is trying to combat type 2 diabetes and/or weight gain.

(8) **Eliminate sugary beverages:** Of course we all know that sodas should be eliminated, however, there are other beverages that are touted as being healthy but will actually worsen diabetes. Sports drinks tend to be advertised as being a somewhat healthy alternative to sodas as they boast electrolytes, but these too are filled with sugars, additives, and artificial ingredients—the costs of these drinks definitely outweigh the benefits. There is much confusion about fruit juices in particular, because we have always been taught that they are good to consume due to the vitamin content. In addition, it is misconception that natural sugar coming from the fruit is unlike processed sugar in terms of the effect it has on our blood sugar. However, our bodies cannot distinguish between the fructose found in fruit from any other types of sugar. Water is the most beneficial beverage whether you have diabetes or are trying to prevent it.

(9) **Eat frequent small meals and snacks if you find yourself hungry:** Eating frequently can help you stay full and fend off hunger or cravings. Incorporating protein and healthy fats in several small meals and snacks all day will help keep blood sugar levels even. If you are awake for sixteen hours per twenty-four-hour day and you eat something every three hours, you will be eating around five times per day. For example, if you are consuming roughly 2,000 calories per day, each small/meal snack will have an average of 400 calories.

Type 2 Diabetes Servings per Day Recommendations		
Food Category	**Servings per Day**	**Food Examples**
Low-Glycemic Vegetables	3–5	Spinach, broccoli, kale, collard greens, cauliflower, cabbage, Brussels sprouts, bok choy, romaine lettuce, arugula
Low-Sugar Fruits	0–1	Tomato, bell pepper, olives, avocado, lemon, raspberries, strawberries, blueberries, blackberries
Probiotic Foods	1–2	Greek yogurt (unsweetened), olives, sauerkraut, tempeh, natto, dark chocolate, kimchi, pickles, cottage cheese
Protein	3–4	Wild salmon, whitefish, shellfish, chicken, eggs, turkey, grass-fed beef, spinach, broccoli, beans, lentils, quinoa, tempeh, natto
Healthy Fats	2–3	Walnuts, macadamia nuts, chia seeds, flax seeds, extra-virgin olive oil, coconut oil, avocado oil, nut butters, wild salmon, sardines, catfish, rainbow trout, herring, oysters, eggs, avocado, seaweed
Caution Foods	0	Bread, pasta, potatoes, rice, cereal, chips, crackers, fast food, fried foods, sugary foods and beverages

Contrary to the above guidelines that help to prevent or manage type 2 diabetes, many doctors still promote meal plans for those with diabetes that contain several daily servings of items such as whole wheat bread, whole wheat pasta, and cereals. These foods will only exacerbate the problem as they will greatly raise your blood sugar despite being whole wheat. So why do doctors still recommend these foods to combat gestational diabetes?

The United States food pyramid that was released in 1992 suggested eating six to eleven servings of grains every day so it has been ingrained (no pun intended) in our society that we need hundreds of gluten-containing carbohydrates to be "healthy." Many medical professionals and nutritionists still base their recommendations on these trends despite the fact that it has been proven that large amounts of these high-glycemic carbohydrates will raise your blood sugar and may lead to type 2 diabetes. These recommendations have been revamped slightly, however, as discussed earlier, the new "MyPlate" still suggests that people eat up to eight slices of bread (or other equivalent grain-containing items) per day! The USDA plays a heavy role in determining these guidelines, and then these same guidelines are incorporated in nutrition education curriculum, which is taught to nutritionists, as well as some doctors. Essentially, as opposed to being based on scientific research and evidence, these recommendations are influenced by food producers, manufactures, and special interest groups. One of the USDA's largest priorities is to strengthen and support food, agriculture, and farming industries, so these guidelines may be disproportionately based on profit as opposed to the health of the general population.

We know it can be nerve-racking to think of possible complications such as type 2 diabetes, and we definitely do not want to alarm you. We bring this condition up since it is becoming more common and the best way to combat it is with knowledge and preventative action. Good nutrition is a very powerful weapon to use; it has been proven, time and again, to greatly reduce the risk of diet-related ailments.

CHAPTER 17
Nutrition Myths That May Be Sabotaging Your Goals

For decades, we have been told to eat particular foods in order to obtain intake from certain vitamins, as well as to achieve specific health and wellness goals. Unfortunately, some of these foods that have been touted as superior sources of the nutrients we need are actually lower quality than what we have been led to believe, due to extensive marketing efforts. The myths we are about to go over stem from general blanket statements that have little to no credible statistics or research to back them up. Unfortunately, these myths—some of which are primary culprits in the deteriorating health of the general population—have spread throughout society as being legitimate and thus are followed by the masses.

Myth ① You need whole wheat bread, pasta, and cereal to get your fiber!

The daily recommended fiber requirement is 25 grams for women and 38 grams for men. Excellent marketing by the food industry has made people believe that whole wheat bread, whole wheat pasta, and whole-grain cereal are good sources of fiber. The truth of the matter is that you can get much more fiber per calorie in other sources of unprocessed, natural foods. Below we compare different food sources of fiber, and illustrate how much one must eat of a particular food to obtain 30 grams of fiber.

Food	Calories Consumed to Reach 30 Grams of Fiber	Carbohydrates Consumed to Reach 30 Grams of Fiber	Sodium Consumed to Reach 30 Grams of Fiber
Whole Wheat Bread	1,350	270g	2025mg
Multigrain Cereal	1,275	275g	2300mg
Whole Wheat Pasta	1,260	246g	20mg
Avocado	702	36g	30mg
Flax Seed	550	30g	30mg
Strawberries	486	117g	6mg
Broccoli	465	90g	450mg
Kale	396	72g	300mg
Chia Seeds	385	33g	13mg
Raspberries	240	56g	4mg
Artichoke Hearts	195	45g	200mg

In addition to having more fiber per calorie, natural foods such as avocado, flax seeds, strawberries, broccoli, kale, chia seeds, raspberries, and artichokes are unprocessed and contain no artificial additives but most commercially made breads, pastas, and cereals do. Whole foods are superior when it comes to vitamins and minerals too. Breads and cereals are fortified with vitamins, which means they do not occur naturally and therefore, they are harder to absorb. The next time you are in a grocery store, look at the ingredient labels of breads, pastas, and cereals—you'll find a plethora of ingredients (such as sugar, high-fructose corn syrup, and preservatives) that are not ideal for weight loss, blood sugar, and overall wellness.

Myth ② Don't eat fish due to environmental toxins!

There are certainly some fish we ought to limit due to high mercury content such as tilefish, shark, and swordfish. On the other hand, there are many types of fish that are extremely beneficial for macro- and micronutrient compositions. Wild salmon, for example, is relatively low in mercury but high in protein and omega-3 fatty acids. As discussed previously, omega-3 fatty acids promote a variety of positive health outcomes such as a lowered risk for heart disease, inflammation, arthritis, and Alzheimer's disease. According to the Natural Resources Defense Council, the following listed seafoods are the lowest in mercury: Anchovies, butterfish, catfish, clam, crab (domestic), crawfish/crayfish, croaker (atlantic), flounder, haddock (atlantic), hake, herring, mullet, oyster, perch (ocean), plaice, pollock, salmon (canned), salmon (fresh), sardine, scallop, shad (American), shrimp, sole (pacific), squid (calamari), trout (freshwater) and whitefish.

Myth ③ Drink lots of milk to get your calcium!

Once again, the marketing for milk has been genius—it does a body good, right? Maybe not so much. First of all, as mentioned earlier, cow's milk has hormones in it that help to grow very large cows! Even if you choose the organic brands, the hormones (intended for cows) still remain. Milk is touted for its calcium content and is known for building strong bones, but some studies suggest that calcium found in cow's milk has no correlation with strong bones and prevention of fractures.[18] Not to mention, at 12 grams of sugar per cup, it's not the ideal beverage for weight loss and blood sugar levels. For more beneficial sources of calcium, please refer to the table below.

Food	Serving	Calories	Calcium (mg)	Sugar (g)
Sardines	3.5 ounce can	210	351	0
Sesame seeds	¼ cup	206	351	0
Collard greens (cooked)	1 cup	49	300	1
Spinach (cooked)	1 cup	41	245	1
Canned salmon	4 ounces	155	232	0
Fresh wild salmon	6 ounces	300	120	0
Kale (raw)	1 cup	33	101	0
Almonds	23 almonds	162	75	1
Broccoli	1 cup	31	74	1.5
Butternut squash	1 cup	63	67	3

---

* You will see in following chapters, that some meals and recipes incorporate canned tuna. If you are one who eats several servings of fish per week and are concerned about mercury intake, we recommend chunk-light tuna since it is three times lower in mercury than solid white albacore.

18 D. Feskanich et al., "Milk, dietary calcium, and bone fractures in women: a 12-year prospective study.," NCBI, June 1997, accessed September 11, 2017, https://www.ncbi.nlm.nih.gov/pmc/articles/PMC1380936/.

Myth ④ Eggs will give you bad cholesterol and put you at risk for heart disease!

Despite eggs being a nutritious whole food, in 1968, the American Heart Association announced that all individuals should eat no more than three eggs per week due to their cholesterol content. Eggs also include invaluable vitamins and minerals, including vitamins B_2, B_5, B_7, B_{12}, and D, as well as omega-3 fats, high-quality protein, choline, iodine, selenium, and zinc. Because eggs contain cholesterol, they have been labeled as an unhealthy food that will contribute to raised LDL (bad) cholesterol and therefore result in putting one at higher risk for heart disease. In 2015, the restriction of egg intake was eliminated from US dietary guidelines, since there is lacking evidence that cholesterol from egg consumption actually causes heart disease. Many mainstream recommendations urge to consume cereal or oatmeal for breakfast due to being "heart healthy" despite the fact that those selections raise blood sugar (while eggs do not), but studies have shown that eating two eggs for breakfast in place of oatmeal reflects no change or increase in biomarkers related to heart disease.[19] In fact, more than fifty years of research has shown that the cholesterol in eggs has very little impact on LDL cholesterol levels, and is not associated with increased cardiovascular disease risk. Moreover, egg intake compensates for an array of common nutritional inadequacies, contributing to overall health and lifespan.[20]

Myth ⑤ You need fortified foods to get your folate!

Folate (otherwise known as B_9) is famously known due to being imperative during pregnancy to prevent neural tube defects, however, folate is extremely important for the rest of the population too. Folate is required to produce red and white blood cells in the bone marrow, create DNA

---

19 Missimer, A., D. DiMarco, C. Andersen, A. Murillo, M. Vergara-Jiminez, and M. Fernandez. "Consuming Two Eggs per Day, as Compared to an Oatmeal Breakfast, Decreases Plasma Ghrelin While Maintaining the LDL/HDL Ratio." NCBI. February 01, 2017. Accessed April 27, 2019. https://www.ncbi.nlm.nih.gov/pmc/articles/PMC5331520/.
20 McNamara, Donald. "The Fifty Year Rehabilitation of the Egg." NCBI. October 2015. Accessed April 27, 2019. https://www.ncbi.nlm.nih.gov/pmc/articles/PMC4632449/.

and RNA, and convert carbohydrates into energy. Synthetic folic acid (the manufactured form of natural folate) is added to a variety of processed foods such as breads, cereals, and pastas, and one of the primary reasons these blood-sugar-raising foods are touted as being healthy is because they contain fortified nutrients such as folic acid. Unfortunately, 40 percent of the population cannot metabolize synthetic folic acid, so consumption of these products may not help you meet your goal of required folic acid intake. There are, however, a large variety of low-carbohydrate whole foods that boast substantial amounts of naturally occurring folate, which is far more bioavailable with higher absorption rates. See below for a chart of folate-rich foods.

Food Source	Serving Size	Folate per Serving (mcg)
Cooked asparagus	1 cup	262
Cooked okra	1 cup	206
Cooked spinach	1 cup	200
Cooked collard greens	1 cup	177
Turnip greens	1 cup	170
Cooked Brussels sprouts	1 cup	160
Raw spinach	1 cup	110
Mustard greens	1 cup	103
Cooked broccoli	1 cup	100
Sunflower seeds	¼ cup	82
Strawberries	8 medium	80
Cooked cauliflower	1 cup	70
Romaine lettuce	1 cup	65
Avocado	½ cup	55
Flax seeds	2 tablespoons	54
Green beans	1 cup	42

Myth (6) You can get everything you need from vitamins!

Synthetic vitamin intake (as opposed to obtaining naturally occurring vitamins from food) has become a popular, quick fix among the general population. Store-bought multivitamins are synthetic versions of real vitamins—they are made in a lab! Typical food intake and the standard American diet lacks essential vitamins and nutrients, which creates the need for the ever-expanding market of fortified nutrients. If you eat a balanced diet of whole foods, you will get what you need for your health and wellness goals. Standard multivitamins are not easily absorbed and contain things like folic acid and ferrous sulfate—inferior versions of folate and iron that have low absorption rates, as well as side effects.

Myth (7) Stay away from fat!

It is true that many fats should be limited, but not all fats are created equal! We tend to overdose on omega-6 fats, which are found in items such as processed foods, vegetable oil, fast food, cookies, chips, and French fries, and then lack the omega-3 fats that are most beneficial for weight loss and heart health. Polyunsaturated omega-3 fats found in foods such as wild salmon, walnuts, flax seed, seaweed, and grass-fed meats are not only beneficial for weight loss and lowered blood sugar levels, they are also associated with the lowering of blood pressure and risk for heart disease. Besides polyunsaturated fats, monounsaturated fats found in extra-virgin olive oil, avocado, and almonds also assist with weight loss, heart disease risk reduction, and inflammation.

Myth (8) You need several servings of whole wheat bread, pasta, and cereal to get your carbs!

Many nutrition resources recommend as much as 325 grams of carbo-hydrates per day, most of which come from gluten-containing foods such as whole wheat bread, pasta, and cereal. These types of carbohy-drates are high glycemic, which means they turn into a lot of sugar! Over-consumption of sugar is one of the primary causes of type 2 diabetes, and the sugar you don't burn off turns to fat, so it is critical to keep sugars and high-glycemic carbohydrates to a minimum. In all actuality, there is absolutely no real nutritional need for carbohydrate consumption to come from breads, pastas, cereals, and crackers, as low-glycemic options such as green vegetables, berries, and avocado, are unprocessed carbohydrate sources that have an abundance of naturally occurring nutrients and fiber.

Myth (9) You need fortified milk, juice, and cereal for vitamin D

Vitamin D intake is critical for tooth and bone health, support of the nervous and immune systems, as well as the brain; it also promotes lung and cardiovascular health and may be associated with cancer prevention. Vitamin D is also one of the most common nutritional deficiencies due to the fact that it can be hard to find in foods. Below you will find a list of foods that have vitamin D, however, if you are one of the millions who are deficient in the vitamin, you may want to consider responsible sun exposure (around 10 to 15 minutes per day with no sunscreen) or consult with your doctor about supplementing.

Sources of Vitamin D

Source	International Units (IU) per Serving
Fish oil	1000
Sockeye salmon (3 ounces)	447
Canned tuna (3 ounces)	154
Some brands of yogurt (6 ounces)	80
Sardines (two whole)	46
Beef liver, cooked (3 ounces)	42
Whole egg (1 large)	41
Swiss cheese (1 ounce)	6

You will receive a lot of advice (good and bad) when it comes to nutrition—hopefully, we have cleared up some confusion for you by dispelling some of these popular myths. Nutrition can be complicated due to the never-ending and conflicting resources that are available in books and on the internet today. As previously mentioned, many aspects of nutrition science have come from funded studies by special interest groups, so it is always best to scratch beneath the surface of some popular myths and recommendations and do your own research.

CHAPTER 18
Mindset Tactics for Achieving Results

Now that you know all about the low-carb protocol, we would like to provide you with some additional tactics for success. Some of these address food intake, while others talk about mental aspects of nutrition and weight loss. In addition, you will find pointers with regard to specific situations where sticking to a food regimen may be more difficult, and ways to overcome nutrition plan slip-ups (which happen to everyone)!

Tactic (1) Find the Way that Works for You

Whether you employ a nutrition plan that has medical-grade weight loss products or not, you will achieve results, so choose the route that is best for you. If you have an extremely busy schedule and you think it would be difficult to give up foods such as pasta, cereal, and cookies, a medical-grade weight loss plan may be the one that makes your transition to the low-carb lifestyle realistic and successful.

Tactic (2) Take It Day by Day

Let's say you want to dive right into the low-carb life but you have a hard-to-kick soda habit, and want to try to give it up cold turkey. If you think in terms of months or weeks or even several days, that can sound overwhelming and maybe even impossible. Take it one day at a time and set a goal for the day. When a goal is very short-term (like 24 hours) it's far easier to reach since it isn't as daunting as thinking long-term.

Tactic ③ Wean off a Bad Habit Slowly

If you can't give up your vice of choice right off the bat, that's totally fine—not many people can! Try weaning off gradually in an attempt to create new habits. Let's get back to the soda as an example, because that obstacle is common for many would-be low-carb dieters. If you drink three sodas per day, simply start by only drinking two sodas per day. That way, the change can be less jarring, as it will happen gradually. After a couple of weeks of two sodas, try to get to one soda or even one-and-a half. After a month or two, maybe you can attempt the day-by-day task of zero sodas!

Tactic ④ Use a Medical-Grade Weight Loss Product as a Cheat Food Substitution

Let's say your big vice is potato chips or chocolate—you can use a specially formulated low-carb, high-protein product as a substitution so you have the same satisfaction without sabotaging your goals. Other cheat foods that Doctors Weight Loss offers in the low-carb form are cookies, wafers, bars, pasta, cereal, puddings, chocolate peanut butter cups, pancakes, and more.

Tactic ⑤ Find More Satisfying Substitutions

Evaluate exactly what you like about a high-carb food and try to replicate some of those favorite tastes with approved foods. For example, you may love potato chips just for the salty taste, so it's possible that other salty foods such as nuts or olives may do the trick. Or if it's the crunch you enjoy from chips and guacamole, some crisp celery, radishes, or jicama dipped in mashed avocado will satisfy the same craving. Pasta can be hard for some to give up, but let's face it, the sauce is usually the flavorful addition that we love about pasta. Try using Alfredo sauce without the noodles—it makes a creamy addition to chicken or zucchini. Nighttime can be hard for those with a sweet tooth—some dark chocolate and a glass of red wine is a low-carb treat that may subside the craving. You can find more substitution ideas in chapter 14!

Tactic ⑥ Find Other Activities to Fill Your Time

It's all too common to eat when not even hungry—usually boredom, sadness, or stress tend to be the main triggers. Finding activities to solve boredom or to use as a coping mechanism can replace the emotional need for food. Taking a walk or jog, getting some errands or household tasks out of the way, relaxing in a bubble bath, finding a good book, or taking up a new hobby are simple ways to replace food as a "thing to do." Physical activity can be the most efficient, as exercise gets the blood pumping and endorphins flowing, causing the feelings of hunger (i.e., sugar cravings) to subside.

Tactic ⑦ Reward Yourself

Some bad nutrition habits are expensive! Let's take alcohol, for example. Happy hour or even some wine at home with dinner certainly adds up. If you abstain from the habit, add up the amount of money you have saved and get yourself something special. Not only will your waistline improve, you'll also enjoy some new clothes or gadgets with all of that money you saved.

Tactic ⑧ Take Charge of Your Social Group

Does your friend group eat out a lot? If so, take charge of *where* your friend group eats, confirming there are healthy choices for you to enjoy as well. Does your friend group drink a lot? If so, plan other social activities that involve physical activity or the outdoors. Explore new options around your area! Also, you may be surprised to find that your friends are interested in adopting new habits as well, so they may welcome the change and suggestions.

Tactic ⑨ Make a Statement

Make sure you are open by sharing with your friends and family about your journey and what changes you are implementing. With regard to celebrations, you can still participate, but take the initiative and bring approved foods such as veggie platters to parties so there is a healthier option. Suggest other home-cooked meals or snacks for others to bring to the party as well! Just as with Tactic 6, being vocal about your goals and newly found lifestyle may inspire others to join you, and it's always more fun to have a buddy.

Tactic (10) Eat Consciously

If you don't want to count calories and macros (it's definitely not required!), a good rule of thumb to follow is to listen to your body and eat consciously. Eating consciously means eating when you are hungry and stopping when you are 80 percent full. It is easier said than done sometimes, but when we eat consciously, we avoid eating out of boredom, stress, or social pressure. Also, it is best to provide focus on your food instead of allocating attention to a book or movie since many tend to overeat while their minds are occupied by something else. If you prefer not to count your calories and macros, that is perfectly fine, but it can be useful to employ this "Seven Scales of Hunger" and try to always hover around level 4.

Seven Scales of Hunger

7. About to burst: Ate way too much food, but it was fun! Same feeling you may experience after Thanksgiving dinner or a birthday party and you think you may never want to see food again.
6. Extremely full: Feeling some discomfort/bloat and need to lie down.
5. Pretty full: Had a few extra bites after being satiated and won't need to eat again for some time.
4. Comfortably satisfied: Ate for fullness and not for fun; stopped when 80 percent full (this is easiest to attain when you eat slowly so your brain has time to signal to your stomach).
3. A tad bit uncomfortable: Didn't eat quite enough (around 70 percent full) and feel a snack (or more) is needed in the near future.
2. Uncomfortable: May have the "growling" sensation in the stomach and or experience low energy.
1. Miserable: Extremely low on energy, unable to focus on tasks, and possibly irritable.

Tactic (11) Control Calories and Portions

Like we have mentioned, counting calories is not required, however, it can be beneficial to have a general idea of how many calories is right for you and your goals, since many people eat far more calories than their bodies need. Despite the fact that the main purpose of food is to fuel our bodies, it is commonly used for comfort, fun, social purposes, and a solution to boredom. Eating proper portions and not until you feel "stuffed" is a key component to achieving and maintaining your ideal weight. The average American is told to consume 2,000 calories per day, but this figure is completely wrong for millions of people. For example, if you are a five-foot, four-inch woman and who wants to weigh 125 pounds, your required intake will range anywhere from 1,400–1,800 calories per day, depending on age and activity level.

Tactic (12) Stick to Your Grocery List and Never Shop While Hungry

Before leaving for the grocery store, make a list and stick to it during your shopping trip. If you don't buy junk food and have it around the house, you are much less likely to eat junk food. The foods found in chapter 2 are all allowed, but of course, you don't need to purchase *all* of them—just your favorites. Always remember to avoid a hungry trip to the grocery store as high-carb foods or extra foods in general may end up in the cart.

Tactic (13) Be Prepared at Work

The workplace is typically a junk food haven. Office donuts, cookies, chips, sodas, and candy vending machines are incredibly tempting, especially when you're hungry. Not to mention, unhealthy snacking may be the majority in your office so the "everybody's doing it" attitude adds to the temptation of giving in. Not being hungry can be the most effective way of combating the food offered in your workplace. It only takes five minutes to put together a convenient snack pack that will keep your hunger satiated and blood sugar levels even. It's as easy as putting a few healthy snacks in your bag the night before work—items like hard-boiled eggs, raw nuts, vegetables and mashed avocado, Greek yogurt, berries, and healthy dinner leftovers.

Tactic (14) Healthy Restaurant Choices

You can still achieve your goals while dining out! If you have a hectic work schedule or you just enjoy eating in restaurants, try to employ the following key concepts when out. For a photo guide of exactly what to eat when dining out, refer to chapter 15.

- Skip the breadbasket—even if it's put in front of you, kindly ask the server to take it away.
- Replace rice, potato, and pasta side dishes with vegetables.
- Use plain oil and vinegar for salad dressing.
- Eliminate pasta and bread-based dishes such as pizza, burgers, and sandwiches; if you order a sandwich or burger, ask your server to lettuce-wrap it (most restaurants will oblige).
- Ask what's in the soup—some have grain-based fillers that you'll want to avoid. Stick to ones made with cream, butter, or avocado bases.
- Ask for any sauces on the side and try to use sparingly.
- Order fresh berries with heavy cream for dessert.
- Avoid waffles, French toast, pancakes, donuts, pastries, or hash browns at breakfast, and opt for egg-based dishes. Keep in mind, eggs Benedict can be made with sliced tomatoes as the base, instead of bread!
- If a restaurant meal is huge (and they usually are), take half of it home and have it for lunch the next day.
- National restaurant chains are required to have nutrition information on-site. Check it out—it may save you a thousand calories!

Tactic (15) Watch Out for Drinkable Sugar

A fruit juice with breakfast, Starbucks Frappuccino in the afternoon, and one soda at dinner add up to almost 900 calories and 100 grams of sugar! People tend to ignore liquid calories and don't realize how easily they result in weight gain. The habit of drinking water is key to losing weight and achieving wellness. Unfortunately, soda and fruit juice have around the same amounts of calories, carbohydrates, and sugar. Even though fruit juice has natural sugar, it's still sugar and sugar, turns into fat if it isn't burned. If you're looking for a good source of vitamin C without the added sugar, opt for items like broccoli, bell pepper, Brussels sprouts, or raspberries.

Tactic (16) Step Off the Wagon—Don't Fall

If you maintain balanced nutrition on a regular basis, then splurging occasionally will not hurt your weight loss goals as long as you return to your good habits immediately after the splurge. Also, if you plan your splurges ahead of time, you will be nutritionally prepared to afford your treat. If you know you're going to a restaurant on Friday night that has your favorite chocolate torte, then be sure to stick to your nutrition plan on Monday, Tuesday, Wednesday, and Thursday, and enjoy your night out on Friday. Once Saturday morning arrives, do not have the "I ruined everything last night, so who cares what I eat today" attitude. Another key concept of weight loss is getting right back on the wagon after taking a controlled step off it.

Tactic (17) Avoid "Train Gain"

If you are one who enjoys exercise, avoid the big mistake of overeating—you will still gain weight, despite the fact you are working out. The average person's workout will only burn around 500 calories, so it is imperative to stick to your nutrition regimen after an exercise session. Too many caloric rewards for a job well done at the gym will backfire and negate all of the hard work you have put in.

We have all heard that people who work out need to "carb up" and eat more calories to have enough energy. This may be true for extremely competitive Ironman triathletes or Olympic athletes but if you're working out like a typical person (jogging eight miles per week or spending six hours per week in the gym), there is no physical need to store away excess carbohydrates to be used for energy. Keep in mind, to lose one pound of weight per week, you must cut out 500 calories from your daily intake. If you spend an hour exercising, you can reach this 500-calorie deficit and your work is done for the day. If you return home from the gym and reward yourself with four slices of pizza (1,300 calories) instead of a sensible 600-calorie meal, you are now in excess of 800 calories. Not working out? Replace a morning scone with two eggs and some blueberries and an afternoon soda with unsweetened iced tea, and there's your 500-calorie deficit!

Tactic (18) Don't Feel Obligated to Exercise to Make a Lifestyle Change

When it comes to weight loss and health improvements, you need to pick and choose your battles. For some, the thought of heading to the gym at 5:00 a.m. before a long day of work prevents many from ever attempting to make a healthy lifestyle change. Fortunately, weight loss and blood sugar improvements are primarily based on good nutrition—working out merely fine-tunes the effort one puts into their daily nutrition plan. If the thought of working out is holding you back from making a change, know that you are not required to exercise to achieve significant results.

Tactic (19) Keep it Simple

The low-carb lifestyle can seem complicated and overwhelming, but it's just a matter of focusing on a few simple concepts. If you take the following steps and implement them into your daily routine, weight loss and wellness will happen for you!

- Stick to your macros—10 to 20 percent carbohydrates, 50 to 60 percent protein, and 20 to 40 percent fat.
- Eliminate or severely limit all high-carb items such as pasta, cereal, rice, potatoes, chips, crackers, pastries, desserts, and sugary beverages.
- Implement medical-grade weight loss products if you think it will be too hard to give up pasta, cereal, cookies, chips, and other high-carb items.
- Use green vegetables and low-sugar fruits as a primary carbohydrate and fiber source.
- Eat healthy fats and high-quality proteins.
- Exercise if possible (but it's not required).
- Make a plan, prepare, and stick to the guidelines.

CHAPTER 19
Doctors Weight Loss
Breakfast Recipes

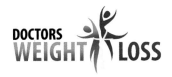

Prosciutto Egg Cups

These egg cups can be made ahead of time and taken on the go for a delicious and low-carb breakfast. For an impressive breakfast or brunch, multiply these ingredients by six, fill a 12-muffin tin, and pair with mixed greens and sparkling mineral water. If prosciutto is not readily available to you, you can replace with deli ham.

SERVES 1 (2 EGG CUPS)

2 eggs

1 scallion, thinly sliced

1 tablespoon unsweetened full-fat coconut milk

Pepper, to taste

1 teaspoon oil

2 large prosciutto slices, folded in half

1. Preheat the oven to 350°F.
2. In a small bowl, beat the eggs and combine with scallions.
3. Mix in the coconut milk and add freshly ground pepper, to taste.
4. Using the oil, grease two muffin tin spaces, and line each cup with one folded prosciutto slice.
5. Using the egg mixture, fill each cup until ⅔ full.
6. Bake for 30 minutes, until eggs are cooked through.

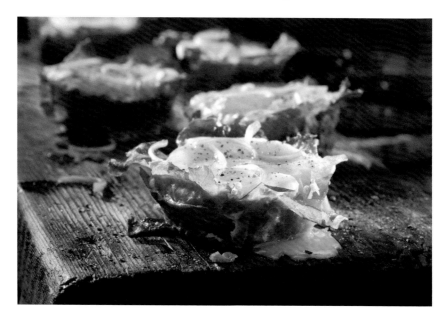

Easy Chia Seed Breakfast Pudding

This only takes minutes to prepare and can be refrigerated overnight if you're looking for a quick breakfast. If you need some added protein and fat, simply pair with a slice or two of bacon.

SERVES 1

½ cup unsweetened coconut milk
1½ tablespoons chia seeds
½ teaspoon vanilla extract
Fresh berries (optional)

1. Combine coconut milk, chia seeds, and vanilla in a small bowl.
2. Cover and refrigerate for at least two hours, or up to overnight.
3. Top with your favorite berries (optional).

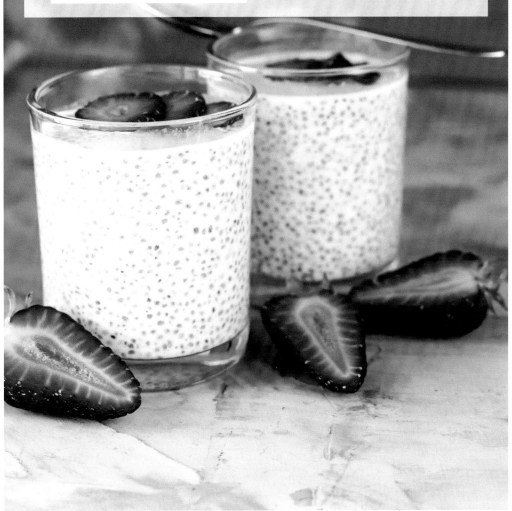

Low-Carb Crepe-Cakes

These crepe-like pancakes are a favorite in the weight-loss community as they are very low in carbohydrates and sugar, while still being very tasty. You can top them with berries, nut butters, bacon crumbles and butter, or salmon and crème fraîche.

SERVES 2

½ cup cream cheese, softened
3 large eggs
3 tablespoons almond flour
Pinch salt (optional)
Pinch cinnamon (optional)
Butter for cooking

1. Place all the ingredients except butter in a blender and blend for 1 minute.
2. Using the butter, cook in a hot pan for 1 minute on each side.

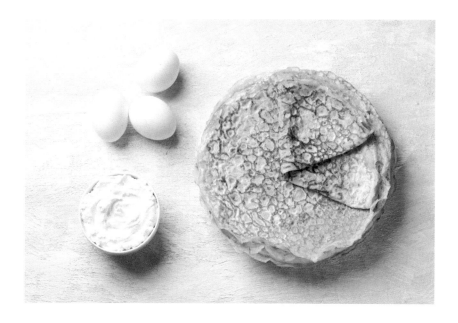

No-Egg Breakfast Bake

Finding high-protein egg alternatives for breakfast can change things up and add variety to your low-carb nutrition plan. You may not commonly find breakfast casserole dishes that are egg-free, but they work nicely for a hearty breakfast. This breakfast bake pairs well with sliced tomatoes drizzled in olive oil and your favorite seasonings.

SERVES 4

2 tablespoons oil, divided
2 large bell peppers of any colors, chopped
Your favorite seasonings
Salt and pepper, to taste
10 ounces turkey or pork breakfast sausage links of your choice
¾ cup grated mozzarella cheese

1. Preheat the oven to 450°F.
2. Use ½ tablespoon oil to grease a medium baking dish.
3. Place chopped peppers into the baking dish, toss with 1 tablespoon oil, and sprinkle with your favorite seasonings, salt, and pepper, and put the dish in the oven and bake 20 minutes.
4. While the peppers cook, heat the rest of the olive oil in a nonstick pan, add the sausages, and cook over medium-high heat until browned on all sides, about 10 to 12 minutes.
5. Remove the sausages and cut into thirds. Once the peppers have cooked for 20 minutes, add the sausages to the dish and bake for an additional 5 minutes.
6. Remove from the oven and turn the oven to broil. Sprinkle the grated cheese over the sausage-pepper combination, put it back in oven, and broil 1 to 2 minutes, or until the cheese is nicely melted and starting to brown. Serve hot.

Eggs in a Hole

A low-carbohydrate take on the old classic, these eggs are encased in bell pepper rings instead of high-glycemic bread. The bell peppers have a wonderful taste and texture, and this dish pairs nicely with either tomatoes or fresh berries.

SERVES 1

1 teaspoon extra-virgin olive oil

2 (½-inch) sliced bell pepper rings

2 eggs

Salt and pepper, to taste

1. In a medium skillet, heat the extra-virgin olive oil over medium heat.
2. Add the bell pepper rings, sauté them on one side for 2 minutes, and then flip over.
3. Crack the eggs into each of the bell pepper rings and reduce the heat to low.
4. Cook the eggs through, about 10 minutes.
5. Add salt and pepper to taste and serve warm, paired with tomatoes or berries.

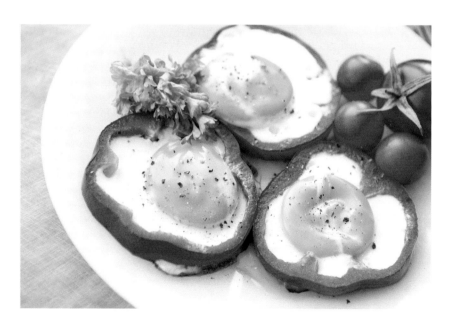

Pizza Eggs

Although this is a low-carbohydrate egg dish, each egg is dressed as its own mini pizza, and it's perfectly circular thanks to the use of a mason jar lid. For added pizza topping flavor, use bell pepper rings (see page 168) instead of mason jar lids to encapsulate the eggs for a perfect mini pizza shape.

SERVES 1

1 tablespoon oil, plus a little extra for greasing
2 large eggs
¼ cup pizza sauce, divided
¼ cup shredded mozzarella, divided
10 mini pepperoni slices
Freshly grated Parmesan, for garnish
Dried oregano, for garnish
Salt and pepper, to taste

1. Heat oil in a medium skillet over medium heat and grease the inside of two mason jar lids. Place the jar lids in the center of the skillet and crack an egg inside each lid.
2. Top each egg with half the pizza sauce, half the cheese, and half the pepperoni slices.
3. Cover with a skillet lid and cook until the egg whites have set and the cheese has melted, 4 to 5 minutes.
4. Top with Parmesan and oregano, season with salt and pepper, and serve.

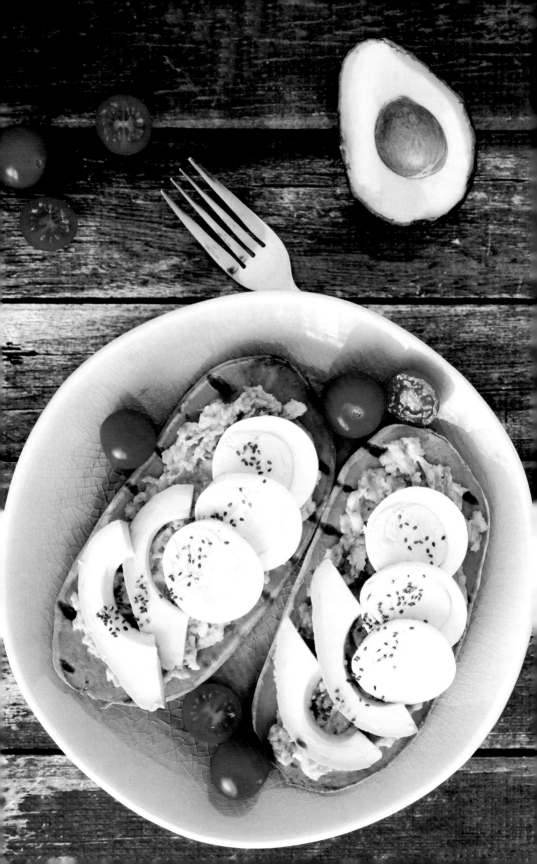

Avocado Sweet Potato "Toast"

While sweet potato is higher in carbohydrates, it boasts so many essential nutrients that it's worth having on a limited basis. This bread-free version of eggs Benedict is very filling. If you're not a fan of eggs, feel free to replace them with sausage for a sweet and savory combination, or with radishes and sprouts for a vegan dish.

1 tablespoon extra-virgin olive oil

1 large sweet potato, sliced into ½-inch planks

Your favorite seasonings

1 avocado, mashed

3 whole eggs

Grape tomatoes, halved, and chives, for garnish (optional)

1. Preheat the oven to 450°F.
2. Toss the sweet potato planks in extra-virgin olive oil and your favorite seasonings; place on a baking sheet.
3. Roast for 15 minutes or until lightly browned and tender, flipping over halfway through.
4. Meanwhile, mash the avocado in a bowl, leaving some small chunks.
5. When the sweet potatoes are 5 to 7 minutes away from being done, poach the eggs or prepare them sunny-side up.
6. When sweet potatoes are finished roasting, plate them and top each plank with avocado mash and 1 egg (replace egg with sprouts and sliced radish for vegan option).
7. Garnish with halved grape tomatoes and chives (optional).

Cottage Cheese Breakfast Bowl

This recipe is super simple, but it's also super delicious and very filling. You only need five minutes to throw these ingredients together to make the perfect pre-work meal. Not to mention, it holds up well in the refrigerator, so it can be packed the night before and taken on-the-go. Not a cottage cheese fan? Simply replace it with plain yogurt.

SERVES 1

¾ cup cottage cheese
1 tablespoon hemp seeds
¼ cup fresh or frozen berries
2 tablespoons crushed almonds

1. Scoop the cottage cheese into a bowl, and top with hemp seeds, berries, and almonds.

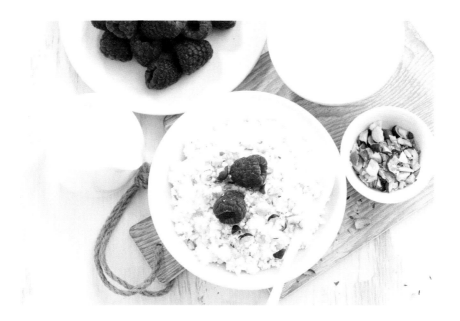

Five-Minute Coffee Cup Biscuits

These fluffy biscuits are made from low-carb ingredients and only take a few minutes to make. Our favorite way to enjoy these is topped with butter or ghee, paired with fresh strawberries, or topped with cream cheese and lox.

SERVES 2 (4 BISCUITS)

1 large egg

3 tablespoons almond flour

1 tablespoon coconut flour

1 tablespoon soft butter

1 tablespoon avocado oil

¼ teaspoon baking powder

Pinch salt

1. Using a fork, thoroughly combine all the ingredients in a microwave-safe mug until the mixture is smooth. Using the back of a spoon, smooth out the top into an even surface.

2. Microwave for 1 minute (depending on your microwave, you may have to slightly alter the time and experiment with high versus medium-high temperatures).

3. Using a potholder or thick cloth, remove the hot mug from the microwave. Cover with a plate and turn upside down, allowing the biscuit to slide out of the coffee cup.

4. Slice into four even pieces. Serve with butter or ghee and sliced strawberries.

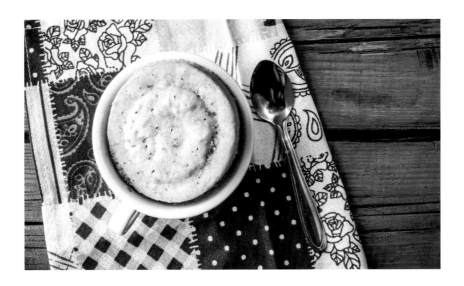

Cream Cheese and Lox Sliders

These cream cheese and lox sliders can be made with just a few ingredients and in two completely different ways. If you're craving more of the traditional bagel with lox you would find in a deli, you can use the biscuits found on the previous page. For a light and refreshing twist, opt for sliced cucumber in place of the biscuits.

SERVES 2 (4 SLIDERS)

3 ounces whipped
    cream cheese
4 Five-Minute Coffee
    Cup Biscuits
    (page 173)
3 ounces wild lox,
    chopped
Fresh dill, for garnish
Capers, for garnish
Freshly squeezed
    lemon, to taste

1. Spread equal amounts of cream cheese on each of the four biscuits.
2. Top each cream cheese biscuit with equal amounts of chopped lox.
3. Garnish each biscuit with fresh dill and capers, and top with a sprinkle of lemon juice.

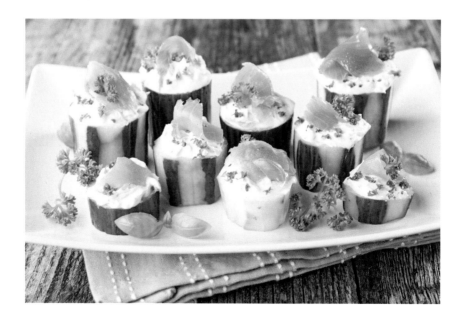

Breakfast Snack Pack

Sometimes you just don't have time to sit down to a hot breakfast, so why not pack it to go? This easy-to-make egg and salmon breakfast box can be put together the night before a busy morning and will ensure that you hit your low-carb macronutrients even on-the-go.

SERVES 1

2 whole eggs

1 tablespoon oil

3–4 asparagus spears

2–3 ounces smoked salmon

1 slice cheese (optional)

Handful raw nuts (optional)

1. Bring water to a boil in a small pot and place the eggs in the pot; boil for 9 minutes for soft- to medium-boiled, or for 12 minutes for hard-boiled.
2. Meanwhile, sauté the asparagus in oil for 6–7 minutes or until tender.
3. Place the eggs, asparagus, and salmon in the meal containers.
4. Add cheese and nuts (optional).

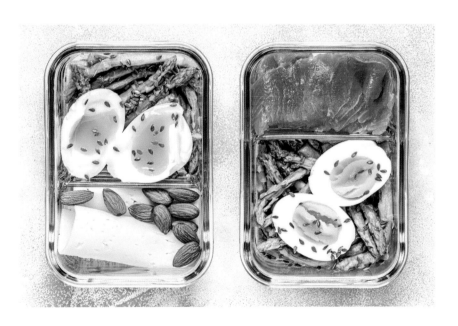

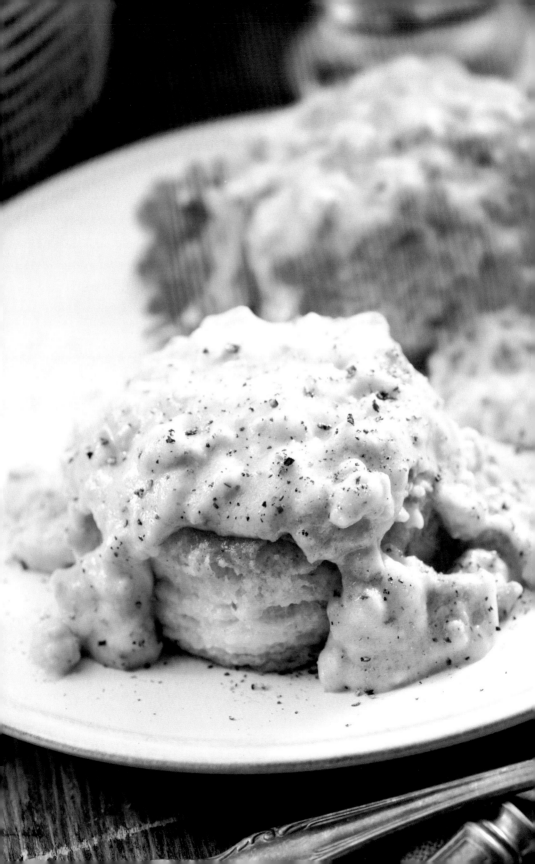

Biscuits and Gravy

Biscuits and gravy isn't a meal that is typically found on the low-carb breakfast menu, but with the Five-Minute Coffee Cup biscuits found in this chapter, you can still enjoy this country favorite. Feel free to pair your biscuits and gravy with eggs or fresh berries.

SERVES 2

4 ounces breakfast
 sausage
3 ounces cream cheese,
 softened
⅓ cup half-and-half
Salt and pepper
4 Five-Minute Coffee
 Cup Biscuits
 (page 173)
Chopped fresh parsley
 for garnish (optional)

1. In a small saucepan over medium heat, brown the sausage while breaking into smaller chunks with a spatula.
2. Add the cream cheese and combine until blended.
3. Add the half-and-half and stir until thoroughly incorporated.
4. Let the gravy reduce over medium heat until it has reached the desired consistency, around 3 to 5 minutes. Remove from the heat and season with salt and pepper, to taste.
5. Pour the gravy over the biscuits and serve warm. Garnish with parsley, if desired.

Grain-Free Breakfast Granola

If you're looking for a cereal replacement that is devoid of grains and filled with protein and healthy fat, grain-free breakfast granola can be topped with your choice of nondairy milk or cream, and berries. You'll have enough left over from this recipe to use the granola as a yogurt topping for another breakfast.

SERVES 3 (½ CUP PER SERVING)

½ cup raw macadamia nuts, chopped

½ cup raw walnuts, chopped

¼ cup cacao nibs

2 tablespoons unsweetened coconut flakes

1 teaspoon vanilla extract

1 teaspoon ground cinnamon

¼ teaspoon salt

2 tablespoons coconut oil, melted

1. Preheat the oven to 325°F.
2. Line a baking sheet with parchment paper.
3. Combine the chopped nuts, cacao nibs, coconut, vanilla, cinnamon, and salt in a medium bowl.
4. Add the coconut oil and mix well.
5. Spread onto the baking sheet and spread evenly into one layer.
6. Bake for 15 minutes or until the granola is toasted at the bottom and fragrant. Keep a close watch and stir frequently as it may burn.
7. Let the granola cool and serve with your favorite nondairy milk.

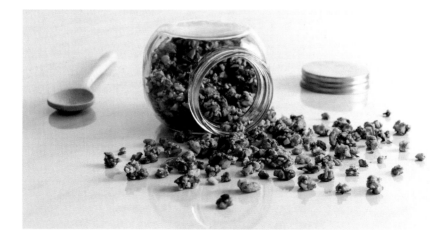

Bacon and Egg Platter

This dish is a bit more delectable and varied compared to the regular bacon-and-eggs breakfast. If you're cooking for a group, simply multiply the recipe and be sure to impress your friends if you're hosting a low-carb Sunday brunch. Garnishing with fresh arugula adds more vitamins and minerals and complements the avocado.

SERVES 1

2 pieces bacon
1 ounce cheese, sliced
½ avocado, sliced
Handful arugula
1 egg

1. Pan-cook the bacon over medium-low heat, turning over every 2 minutes, until cooked through, about 10 minutes.
2. While the bacon is cooking, plate the cheese, avocado, and arugula.
3. Plate the bacon. Add the egg to the hot bacon grease and cook through, about 5 minutes.

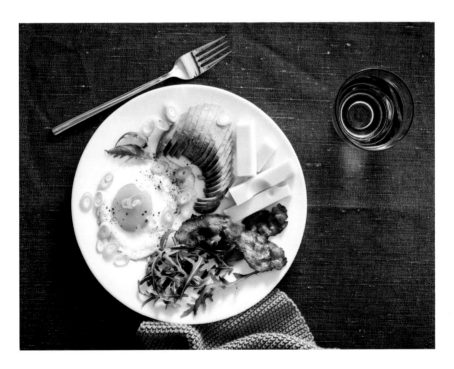

CHAPTER 20

Doctors Weight Loss
Lunch Recipes

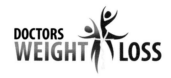

Spicy Mayonnaise Ahi Poke Bowl

Preparing a sashimi-inspired dish at home can seem intimidating, but it's actually super simple. The key is to find high-quality and fresh sushi-grade fish, so check your local health food grocery that has a reputable seafood counter. After that, it's just a matter of chopping and mixing a few ingredients.

SERVES 2

½ pound sushi-grade ahi
tuna, cubed

¼ cup mayonnaise

1 tablespoon sriracha

1 avocado, cubed

½ zucchini, thinly sliced into
ribbons

¼ cup scallions, sliced, optional

1 tablespoon black and/or
white sesame seeds

1. Place the tuna in a medium mixing bowl.
2. Combine the mayonnaise and sriracha to make the spicy mayonnaise. Pour over the tuna and gently toss to coat.
3. Add the rest of the ingredients and gently toss to combine. Serve cold.

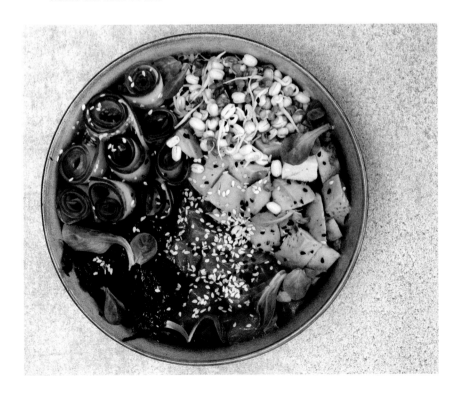

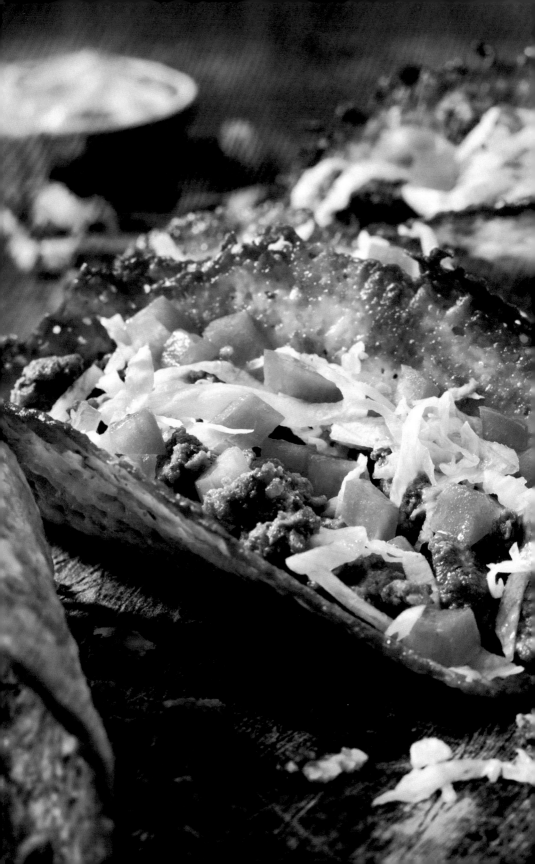

Cheese Shell Tacos

If you like your tacos with that crunchy chip-like shell, this dish is definitely for you. Just using one low-carb ingredient (cheese) and a simple baking technique will give you crunchy taco shells with even more cheesy flavor. This base recipe is just the foundation for an array of possibilities for different proteins, sauces, seasonings, and toppings.

MAKES 6 TACOS

2 cups shredded cheddar cheese
½ pound ground beef
1 tablespoon sugar-free taco seasoning
¼ cup water

Topping Suggestions

2 cups shredded lettuce
1 medium tomato, diced
⅓ cup diced yellow onions
1 avocado, sliced or mashed
½ cup sour cream
Fresh cilantro, to taste

1. Preheat the oven to 375°F and line two baking sheets with parchment paper.
2. Divide the cheese into 6 small piles on your prepared baking sheets, with plenty of space in between so the shells do not run together.
3. Bake for 7 to 10 minutes, until the edges start to brown and the cheese is no longer runny.
4. Meanwhile, prop up one wooden spoon or two kabob skewers (spaced 1 inch apart) with two cups or cans.
5. Remove the melted cheese round from the oven, and, while the cheese is still flexible, drape it over the wooden spoon handle or skewers, letting it harden until cool. Repeat the process with all the cheese rounds.
6. In a medium skillet, brown the ground beef and drain the fat. Add the taco seasoning and water, stirring well. Bring to a simmer, and reduce for 3 to 5 minutes.
7. Remove the ground beef from the heat and fill each cheese shell. Garnish with toppings of choice.

Lunch Snack Pack

Sometimes you don't feel like an actual meal for lunch, and a variety of delicious snacks will do the trick—not to mention, this can be easier and faster to pack and take on the go. For a full week of lunches, simply multiply this recipe by five, package, and refrigerate, as it will all hold up for the week.

SERVES 1

1 small container Greek yogurt

4 strawberries

¼ cup raw walnuts

Handful raw broccoli florets and celery sticks

½ cup mashed avocado for dipping

2 tablespoons peanut butter for dipping

1 hard-boiled egg

1. Package all the ingredients in a portable container and refrigerate.

Easy Pistachio Avocado Salad

This salad does well on its own, but if you're looking for more protein, chicken is a great addition. The fats from nuts, seeds, avocado, and oil will help you hit your low-carb macros in the healthiest way possible, and if you prefer to batch prepare this so you have several servings for the week, simply sub kale in for the romaine, as it stands up better after a few days in the fridge.

SERVES 2

Salad:
1 head romaine lettuce, chopped
¼ cup sliced red onions
½ cup shelled pistachio halves
¼ cup shelled hemp seeds
1 avocado, sliced

Dressing:
2 tablespoons extra-virgin olive oil
1 tablespoon apple cider vinegar
1 tablespoon coconut aminos
Freshly squeezed lemon, to taste

1. Place the chopped romaine in a large bowl.
2. Add the scallions, pistachios, hemp seeds, and avocado.
3. Whisk all the dressing ingredients and thoroughly toss the dressing with the salad.

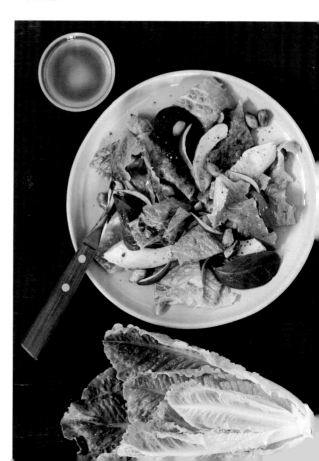

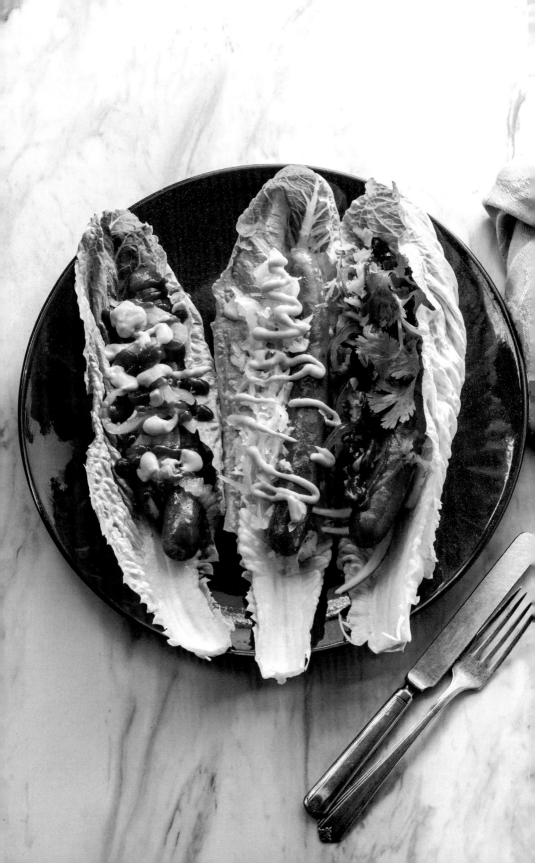

Low-Carb Hot Dogs Your Way

We don't recommend too many meals of hot dogs (or deli meats), but if only consumed occasionally, they won't sabotage your wellness goals. This hot dog dish has a delicious combination of flavors, making your standard high-carb hot dog seem a bit boring. You won't even miss the bun!

SERVES 1

2 nitrate-free hot dogs
2 large romaine lettuce
    leaves
2 tablespoons
    sauerkraut
1 tablespoon sliced red
    onion
2 tablespoons grated
    cheddar cheese
Ketchup and mustard,
    to taste

1. Grill or boil the hot dogs until warmed through.
2. Place each hot dog on a romaine lettuce leaf.
3. Top one hot dog with sauerkraut and mustard.
4. Top the other hot dog with onion, cheese, ketchup, and mustard.

Bell Pepper Nachos

Triangular bell pepper slices can be used as low-carbohydrate tortilla chips and with all of the nacho toppings, this dish tastes just like the classic. This base recipe can be modified to add any of your favorite nacho toppings, and the flavors will be sure to quench any Mexican food cravings, and with zero guilt!

SERVES 2–3

4 large bell peppers
(assorted colors)
1 pound ground beef
3 tablespoons low-sugar
taco seasoning
⅔ cup beef broth
1½ cups shredded
cheese

Optional Toppings
½ cup diced tomatoes
⅓ cup diced scallions
½ cup mashed avocado
⅓ cup sour cream
Cilantro, to taste

1. Preheat the oven to 375°F. Remove the membranes from the bell peppers and cut them into triangle slices. Place the slices on a baking sheet and bake for 10 minutes until tender.
2. While the peppers are roasting, brown the ground beef in a skillet over medium heat and drain the excess liquid.
3. Add the taco seasoning and beef broth and bring to a boil. Simmer over medium heat for about 5 minutes, or until it has reduced, leaving little to no liquid.
4. Spoon the ground beef on the bell pepper slices and top with the grated cheese. Return the baking sheet to the oven for 5 to 6 minutes, until the cheese has melted.
5. Remove from the oven and add the optional toppings of choice.

Zucchini Boat Tuna Salad

This is a healthier version of traditional mayonnaise-filled tuna salad, and the handheld zucchini boats are convenient for a picnic or work lunch. This simple recipe is high in protein, low in carbohydrates, high in healthy fat, and only takes minutes to prepare.

SERVES 1

1 large zucchini
1 can tuna packed in
    water (strain as much
    water as possible)
1 tablespoon avocado oil
    mayonnaise
Juice of ½ lemon
¼ bell pepper, diced
Handful of parsley,
    chopped
Black pepper, to taste

1. Hollow out the zucchini by scraping out the inner soft layer and set aside.
2. Mix the tuna with the mayonnaise, the lemon juice, and the bell pepper.
3. Fill the zucchini boat with tuna mixture and top with parsley and ground pepper.

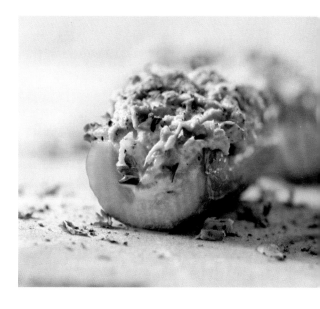

Wine Country Lunch Platter

Sometimes it's nice to change it up and have a smorgasbord platter as opposed to a standard hot meal. This is the perfect lunch to introduce your new low-carb lifestyle to your friends—and you can even enjoy a glass or two of red wine with it!

SERVES 1

4 ounces cooked pork chop, sliced

½ cup chopped or sliced cucumber

1 egg, soft-boiled, halved

1 ounce cheese, sliced

5 olives

1 ounce nuts

¼ cup berries (optional)

1. Arrange all the ingredients on a platter.
2. Serve with a glass of pinot noir or sauvignon if desired.

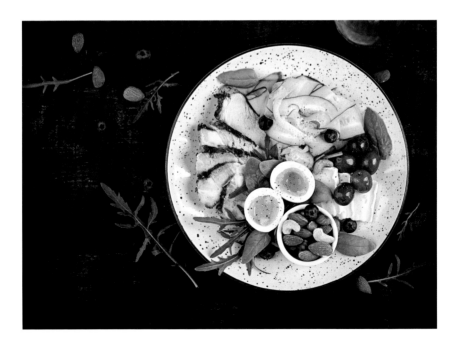

Minute No-Bake Chicken Cauliflower Cheese Casserole

If you're in a rush, this no-bake (and no-stove) casserole is a delicious combination of chicken, cauliflower, and cheese. To batch-cook, simply triple the recipe and refrigerate for up to one week or freeze for up to three months. Pair with grilled asparagus or a small side salad.

SERVES 6

1 pound cauliflower rice
1½ tablespoons water
4 ounces sour cream
1 cup cheddar cheese, shredded
1 pound packaged rotisserie chicken (already cooked)
3 tablespoons chives
4 tablespoons butter
1 cup Parmesan cheese
2 teaspoons garlic
Salt and pepper, to taste

1. Place the cauliflower in a microwave-safe dish with the water. Cover with a piece of plastic wrap, leaving a small gap to let air release.
2. Microwave on high heat for 3 minutes or until tender.
3. Drain excess water from the cauliflower and place it in a large microwave-safe bowl; mix in all other ingredients.
4. Microwave again on high for 90 seconds and mix again.

Egg Roll in a Bowl

This dish gives you all of the delicious fillings found in an egg roll, in one big bowl. These bowls keep really well in the refrigerator, so this is a great recipe to batch cook ahead of time so you have tasty Chinese-inspired flavors for the week.

SERVES 2–3

1 pound ground chicken or pork sausage

1 teaspoon minced ginger

3 tablespoons soy sauce

1½ teaspoons sesame oil

4½ cups packaged coleslaw mix (shredded cabbage and carrots)

3 scallions, chopped

1. Brown the meat in a medium nonstick skillet until cooked all the way through and then add the ginger.
2. Add soy sauce and sesame oil.
3. Add the coleslaw and stir until coated with sauce.
4. Add the scallions and mix thoroughly.

Low-Carb Greek Platter

This hearty Greek platter includes a variety of popular Mediterranean foods without packing in the carbohydrates, and we promise you won't miss the pita bread! All components of this dish hold up well in the refrigerator, so simply double the recipe to batch cook.

SERVES 2

1 tablespoon oil
¾ pound chicken, cubed
Your favorite
    seasonings, to taste
1 small cucumber,
    chopped
10 grape tomatoes,
    halved
¼ cup thinly sliced red
    onion
10 kalamata olives,
    halved
½ cup crumbled feta
    cheese
½ cup tzatziki
    (page 253)

Dressing:
¼ cup extra-virgin olive
    oil
1 tablespoon red wine
    vinegar
Dollop Dijon mustard
Dried oregano, to taste
Salt and pepper, to taste

1. In a pan with oil over medium-high heat, cook the chicken on one side until brown, about 4 minutes. Add your favorite seasonings and turn over. Continue to cook until done, around 4 minutes, flipping occasionally.
2. Meanwhile, add the cucumber, tomatoes, onion, olives, and feta cheese to a medium bowl and toss.
3. Whisk all dressing ingredients until thoroughly combined. Pour over the salad and toss until coated.
4. Plate the chicken, salad, and tzatziki, and serve.

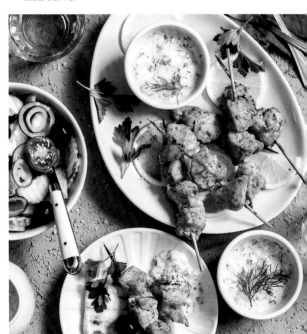

Chicken and Broccoli Alfredo

This dish can be used interchangeably for lunch or dinner, but we included it here because it can be easily packed for lunch and reheated. You won't miss the pasta in this decadent dish, and if you want to make it really fast and simple, use precooked rotisserie chicken.

SERVES 4

1 tablespoon butter

½ cup yellow onions, chopped

2 cloves garlic, pressed

1 cup white mushrooms, sliced

1 pound chicken breasts or thighs, cooked and cubed

3 cups broccoli florets, steamed

1½ cups Alfredo sauce (page 252) or store-bought

½ cup shaved Parmesan cheese

1 tablespoon fresh parsley, chopped (optional)

1. In a large skillet, melt the butter over medium heat. Add the onions, garlic, and mushrooms. Cook until the onions are translucent and the mushrooms are tender.
2. Add the chicken, broccoli, and Alfredo sauce, and combine until evenly coated.
3. Simmer for 3 to 4 minutes, stirring occasionally.
4. Divide among 4 bowls or sealed containers (if storing for work lunches) and garnish with Parmesan cheese and parsley (optional) before serving.

Deluxe Vegan Protein Bowl with Tahini Dressing

This high-protein vegan bowl is a mixture of sweet and savory and will give you healthy fats, low-glycemic carbohydrates, and several vitamins and minerals, in addition to plant-based protein. If you're not vegan, grilled chicken makes an excellent addition.

SERVES 2

For the Bowl:

1 cup broccoli florets

1 cup cubed butternut squash

1 tablespoon extra-virgin olive oil

Salt and pepper, to taste

Garlic powder, to taste

2 cups curly kale or arugula

Handful shredded purple cabbage

½ avocado, sliced

1 tablespoon hemp seeds

1 tablespoon sesame seeds

Tahini Dressing:

¼ cup tahini

Juice of 1 lemon

1 clove garlic, minced

Salt and pepper, to taste

1–2 tablespoons warm water, to thin

Dash of real maple syrup (optional)

1. Preheat the oven to 400°F.
2. Toss the broccoli and cubed butternut squash in olive oil, salt, pepper, and garlic powder, and place on a baking sheet.
3. Roast for 25 to 30 minutes or until tender.
4. Meanwhile, place the kale or arugula in a medium bowl.
5. Top with the cabbage, avocado, broccoli, and roasted butternut squash.
6. Combine all dressing ingredients thoroughly and drizzle on top.
7. Top with hemp seeds and sesame seeds.

Loaded Cauliflower Salad

If you love potato salad, this will do the trick without all of the unwanted carbohydrates. Typically, potato salad is used as a potluck side dish, but this loaded version will stand up on its own as a satisfying meal. If you feel like you need some more protein, pair with some grilled chicken or steak.

SERVES 3

4 slices bacon

1 head cauliflower, chopped into bite-size pieces

2 tablespoons extra-virgin olive oil

2 cloves garlic, minced

Salt and pepper, to taste

½ cup full-fat Greek yogurt

½ cup avocado oil mayonnaise

4 ounces shredded sharp white cheddar cheese

4 scallions, chopped

1 bunch chopped fresh chives

2 dashes hot pepper sauce

¼ teaspoon paprika

1. Place the bacon in a medium skillet and cook over medium heat, while turning over occasionally for 10 minutes, or until cooked through to your liking. Chop into small bits and set aside.

2. Preheat the oven to 400°F, and line a baking sheet with foil.

3. Combine the cauliflower, extra-virgin olive oil, garlic, salt, and pepper in a large bowl. Spread the cauliflower evenly on the lined baking sheet, and roast for 15 to 20 minutes or until lightly browned.

4. Place the roasted cauliflower, Greek yogurt, and mayonnaise in a large bowl and stir until cauliflower is evenly coated.

5. Fold in the bacon bits, shredded cheese, scallions, chives, hot sauce, and paprika. Add more salt and pepper, to taste.

6. Refrigerate for at least 2 hours before serving.

Parmesan Kale Salad

This universal salad base pairs nicely with most flavors. The avocado dressing is simple and healthy, and provides a creamy texture that is reminiscent of more decadent salad dressings that don't have the most ideal ingredients. Hard-boiled eggs or chopped steak are complementary additions.

SERVES 1

2 cups curly kale or
  chopped romaine
  lettuce
½ avocado
2 tablespoons oil
1 teaspoon apple cider
  vinegar
1–2 tablespoons grated
  Parmesan cheese
Freshly squeezed
  lemon, to taste
Pine nuts (optional)

1. Place the greens in a medium bowl.
2. In a small bowl, mash the avocado with a fork until you have a paste texture.
3. Drizzle in the oil gradually as you thoroughly combine with the avocado.
4. Drizzle in the vinegar and thoroughly combine.
5. Using your hands, massage the dressing into the greens until all leaves are coated.
6. Top with Parmesan cheese, freshly squeezed lemon, and pine nuts (optional).

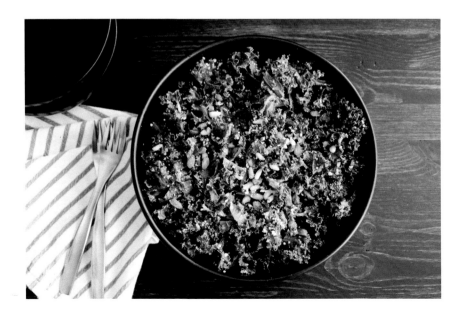

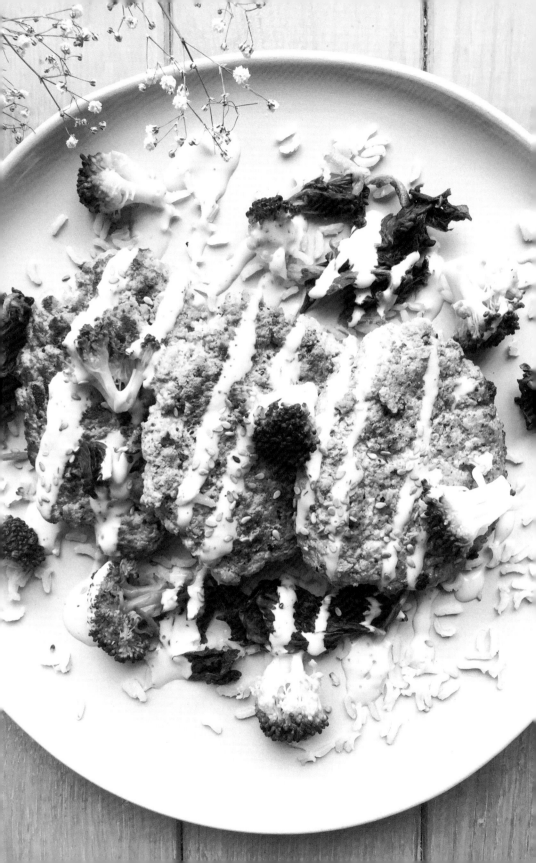

Tuna Burgers

Crab cakes are delicious,—but they can be expensive and difficult to make. These easy (and inexpensive!) tuna burgers are reminiscent of your favorite seafood restaurant's crab cakes but can be made in a snap and with ingredients found in the kitchen pantry. Avocado oil mayonnaise and whole-grain mustard make great low-carb dips for your tuna burgers.

SERVES 4

2 (5-ounce) cans solid white albacore tuna in oil

2½ tablespoons almond flour

2 tablespoons mayonnaise

1 large egg, beaten

½ tablespoon olive oil or avocado oil

Salt and pepper, to taste

Optional:

Chopped scallions, to taste

Capers, to taste

1. In a medium bowl, combine all the ingredients (including optional ingredients), except the oil. Mix until thoroughly combined.
2. Form the mixture into 4 patties, around ¾-inch thick.
3. In a large pan, heat the oil over medium-high heat. Place the patties in the pan.
4. Cook the patties on one side for 4 to 5 minutes, or until they have set and are golden on one side.
5. Flip the patties over and cook for 4 to 5 minutes.
6. Serve warm, or store in the refrigerator in an airtight container with parchment paper to separate the patties.

British Bangers and Mash

Yes, we do advise to limit processed meats, but if you're in a pickle for a quick lunch, this is a great option. Not to mention, I thought I would pay homage to my British roots with this one! A tip is to quadruple the mashed cauliflower recipe so you have the tasty low-carb side dish on hand in your refrigerator.

SERVES 1

1 cup cauliflower florets
2 hots dogs or sausages
¼ cup grated Parmesan cheese
Salt and pepper, to taste
Mustard, to garnish (optional)
Sauerkraut, to garnish (optional)

1. Steam the cauliflower over medium-high heat until extremely tender, about 20 minutes.
2. Meanwhile, prepare the hot dogs or sausages according to package directions.
3. Once the cauliflower is steamed, mashed it in a medium bowl with the grated Parmesan, salt, and pepper until thoroughly combined.
4. Plate the hot dogs or sausages with the mashed cauliflower and garnish (optional).

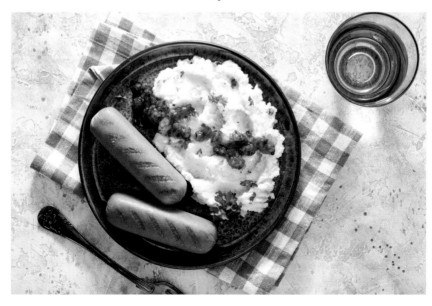

Easy Lunch Time
Roasted Cheesy Chicken

We usually don't have time to prepare a nice roasted chicken dish for lunch, but this recipe is so easy, you can whip it up in only five minutes. Not to mention, the flavors are unique to most poultry dishes so it's not only simple, but also different. Pair this decadent fare with a simple side salad or your favorite roasted veggies for a complete meal.

SERVES 4

½ cup grated or
    shredded Parmesan
    cheese
1 cup mayonnaise
1 teaspoon garlic
    powder
1½ teaspoons salt
½ teaspoon pepper
4 chicken breasts

1. Preheat the oven to 375°F. Line a baking sheet with aluminum foil or parchment paper.
2. Excluding the chicken breasts, combine all other ingredients in a medium bowl.
3. Using a spoon, spread the mixture over each chicken breast.
4. Bake for 45 minutes, and serve warm.

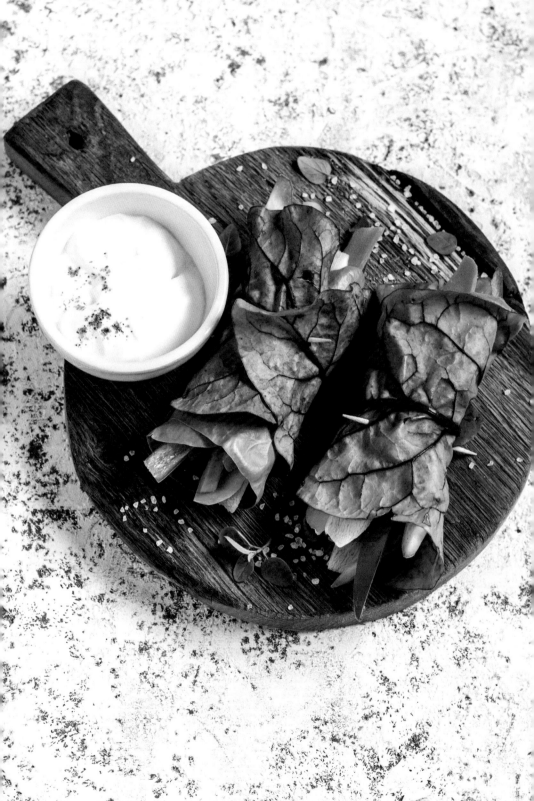

Mediterranean Swiss Chard Wrap

This low-carb wrap is a refreshing change a pace! This base recipe can be built upon with lots of colorful produce and dipping sauces. Or if you are looking for more protein, diced chicken or steak makes a tasty addition.

SERVES 1

2 tablespoons full-fat plain yogurt
2 tablespoons crumbled feta cheese
2 tablespoons pitted, chopped olives
¼ ripe avocado, diced
2 large Swiss chard leaves
4 thin slices bell pepper (any colors)
Salt and pepper, to taste

1. In a large bowl, mash the yogurt, feta, olives, and avocado into a chunky paste. Season with salt and pepper and set aside.
2. Place the Swiss chard leaves on a cutting board and using a knife, remove the stems and around 2 inches of the spine from each leaf.
3. Divide the yogurt mixture in half and spoon into each leaf. Place the sliced bell pepper on the mixture and roll into a wrap. Secure with a toothpick.
4. To form a burrito-style wrap, place a horizontal mound of mixture on the lower third of each leaf, just above the area where the spine was removed, and add the bell pepper slices. Fold in the two vertical ends of one leaf and roll from the bottom. Secure with a toothpick.
5. Repeat with the second wrap and enjoy cold.

CHAPTER 21

Doctors Weight Loss
Dinner Recipes

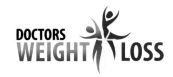

Cheesy Ground Beef and Green Bean Casserole

This high-protein comfort food dish tastes like Grandma's home cooking, and you won't notice the missing carbohydrates. For versatile dish, you can replace the ground beef with ground or bite-size chicken or pork, and it pairs well with a crisp salad.

SERVES 6

1 pound ground beef

3 ounces cream cheese

½ cup beef broth

½ cup heavy cream

2 teaspoons coconut aminos

1 teaspoon garlic powder

½ teaspoon salt

½ teaspoon pepper

2 cans green beans, drained

¾ cup shredded cheddar cheese

¾ cup shredded mozzarella cheese

1. Preheat the oven to 350°F.
2. Brown the ground beef in a medium skillet and drain the excess grease.
3. Add the cream cheese and stir until melted. Then add the beef broth, cream, coconut aminos, garlic powder, and salt and pepper.
4. Bring to a boil and cook on a simmer, about 15 minutes.
5. Once the ground beef mixture thickens, add the 2 cans of drained green beans on top.
6. Sprinkle all of the shredded cheese on top of the green beans, transfer the skillet to the oven, and bake for 25 minutes.

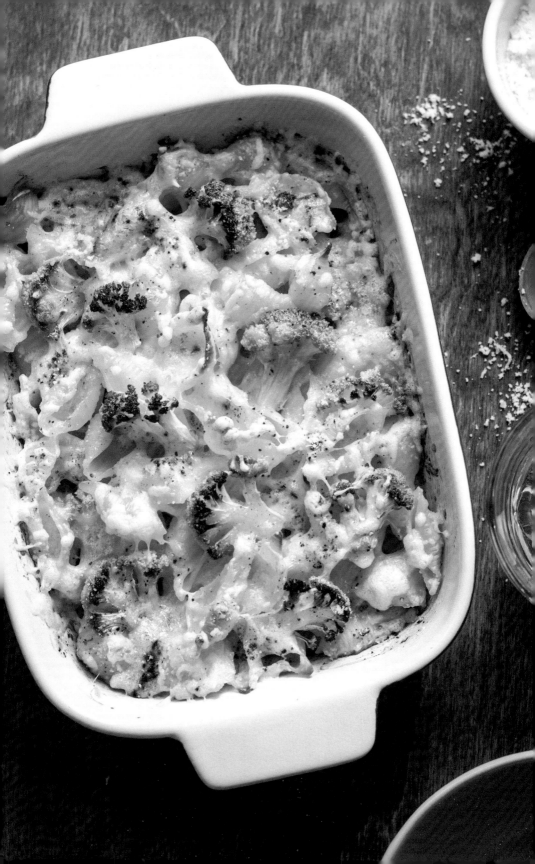

Low-Carb Cauliflower Mac N' Cheese

Mac n' cheese is probably one of the greatest known comfort foods, and you can still work it in while being low-carb. While the actual pasta is missing, the flavor and extreme cheesiness is still there—and if you're looking for more protein, simply pair with a steak or chicken breast to make it extra filling.

SERVES 8

Butter, for baking dish
2 medium heads cauliflower, cut into florets
2 tablespoons avocado oil
Salt, to taste
1 cup heavy cream
6 ounces cream cheese, cubed
4 cups shredded cheddar cheese
2 cups shredded mozzarella cheese
¼ cup grated Parmesan cheese
Freshly ground pepper, to taste
Fresh parsley, chopped (for garnish)

1. Preheat the oven to 375°F and butter a 9x13-inch baking dish.
2. In a large bowl, toss the cauliflower florets with the oil and season to taste with salt. Spread cauliflower on two baking sheets and roast until lightly golden, about 40 minutes.
3. While the cauliflower is roasting, heat the cream in a large pot over medium heat. Bring up to a simmer and then decrease heat to low and stir in all cheeses except the Parmesan until melted and combined.
4. Remove from the heat and season with ground pepper (and additional salt) as needed.
5. Fold the cheese mixture into the roasted cauliflower and transfer the mixture to the prepared baking dish.
6. Bake for about 15 minutes or until golden brown. Top with grated Parmesan and bake for an additional 2 minutes.
7. Garnish with chopped parsley and serve.

Slow Cooker Creamy Bacon Chicken

If you're tired of basic chicken recipes, you may want to try this as it's gooey and cheesy, with bacon added. This dish is filling on its own or can be paired with a crisp green salad, and the best part is, that it's extremely low-carb!

SERVES 6

½ cup bone broth or chicken stock

1 tablespoon dried parsley

2 teaspoons dried dill

1 teaspoon dried chives

½ teaspoon onion powder

¼ teaspoon garlic powder

2 pounds boneless, skinless chicken breasts

Salt and pepper, to taste

16 ounces cream cheese, cubed

2¼ cups shredded cheddar cheese, divided

8 slices cooked bacon, crumbled

Chopped chives, for serving

1. Pour the chicken broth into a slow cooker and add parsley, dill, chives, onion powder, and garlic powder.
2. Add half the chicken and season with salt and pepper, to taste. Repeat with the remainder of the chicken.
3. Stir the broth to coat the chicken and set the slow cooker on low for 6 hours or on high for 2 hours.
4. When done, use two forks to shred the chicken while it remains in the slow cooker. Stir in the cream cheese and 2 cups of the shredded cheddar until melted.
5. To serve, top with remaining cheddar cheese, bacon, and chives.

Classic Cheeseburger in a Bowl

If you're missing a good old drive-through burger, this dish will not disappoint. You'll get all of the classic taste and flavors from your favorite fast-food order, even down to the sauce!

SERVES 3

For the Bowl:

1 pound ground beef
½ cup yellow onion, diced
Salt and pepper, to taste
6 cups iceberg or romaine
　　lettuce, shredded
½ cup sliced red onion
1 cup shredded cheddar
　　cheese
1 cup tomato, diced
　　(optional)
¼ cup dill pickles, sliced or
　　diced

For the Sauce:

¾ cup mayonnaise
2 tablespoons dill pickles,
　　finely minced
1 tablespoon Thousand
　　Island dressing or
　　mustard
½ teaspoon smoked
　　paprika
½ teaspoon garlic powder
½ teaspoon onion powder

1. Add the beef to a large pan and brown over medium-high heat for 3–4 minutes, breaking up the beef into crumbles.
2. Add the yellow onion, salt, and pepper, and continue to cook for 4 to 5 minutes or until the onion is softened and the beef is browned, and cooked through.
3. Meanwhile, whisk all sauce ingredients in a medium bowl until combined.
4. Divide lettuce into 3 bowls, top each bowl with ⅓ of the browned beef, onion, cheese, tomato (optional), and pickles.
5. To serve, drizzle with the special sauce.

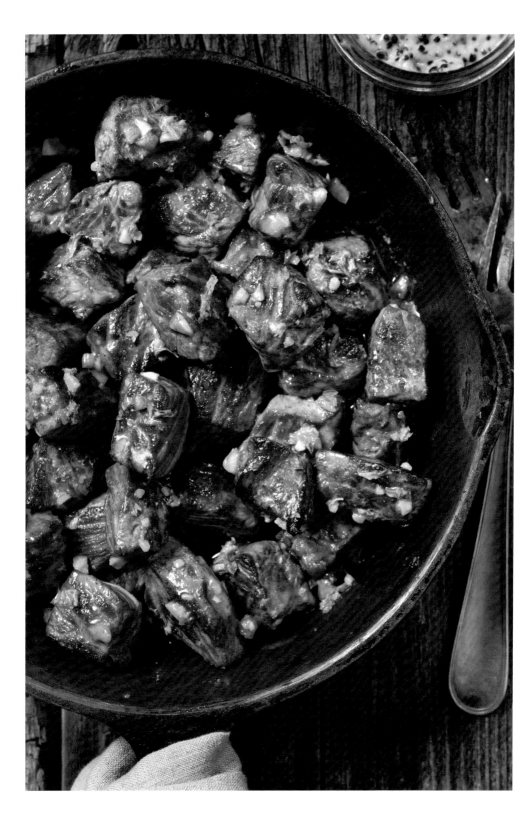

Garlic Butter Steak Bites

This is a unique and simple way to prepare you steak, and so many variations can be created from this easy base recipe by adding your own seasonings and flavors. Steak bites are delicious with a trio of dips—mashed avocado, avocado oil mayonnaise, and tzatziki (page 253) are our favorites, or you can pair with a side salad with ranch dressing.

SERVES 3–4

2 pounds rib eye steak

Salt and pepper, to taste

4 tablespoons oil, divided

4 tablespoons butter, divided

2 large garlic cloves, minced and divided

1 teaspoon fresh parsley leaves, minced

1. Cut steak into ¾-inch cubes and season with salt and pepper.
2. Heat half of the oil in a large skillet over medium-high heat. Add half the steak in a single layer and cook, turning a few times until golden and medium rare, about 5 minutes.
3. Add half of the butter and half of the garlic and toss to coat.
4. Remove the steak to a serving bowl. Repeat with the remaining steak.
5. Garnish steak with parsley.

Rosemary Goat Cheese and Mushroom Stuffed Pork Chops

If you're looking for a pork chop dish that is a bit more fancy and flavorful, but doesn't require lots of ingredients, this meal can be used for an easy dinner at home or even to host a gathering. For a pop of flavor, pair the stuffed chops with some cold and crisp sauerkraut.

SERVES 2

½ cup chopped white mushrooms

2 ounces goat cheese, crumbled

1 teaspoon rosemary, freshly chopped or dried

1 large garlic clove, pressed

2 (12-ounce) bone-in pork chops (1-inch thick)

Salt and pepper, to taste

1 tablespoon oil

1. Preheat the oven to 350°F.
2. In a small bowl, gently combine the mushrooms, goat cheese, rosemary, and garlic.
3. Cut a large slit in the side of each pork chop to make a pocket for the filling. Do not pierce the back or sides of the chops so the filling does not spill out.
4. Stuff the pork chops with the goat cheese filling and press closed. Season the pork chops with salt and pepper, to taste.
5. Heat the oil in a large oven-safe skillet over medium-high heat. Add the stuffed chops and sear until golden brown, 2 to 3 minutes per side.
6. Transfer the skillet to the oven and cook for 25 to 30 minutes until the internal temperature of the chops reaches 145°F. Allow them to rest for 3 minutes before serving.

Spinach, Artichoke, Asparagus Stuffed Chicken

This is a favorite of many low-carb dieters, and it's a very family-friendly way to get some veggies in the meal. For an interesting seafood dish, just follow the same instructions but use two thick salmon fillets instead of chicken. This is a complete low-carb meal, or it can be served with a crisp side salad.

SERVES 2

2 chicken breasts

4 tablespoons store-bought spinach artichoke dip, divided

6 asparagus spears

Salt and pepper, to taste

1. Preheat the oven to 350°F.
2. Butterfly the chicken breasts and spread 2 tablespoons of spinach artichoke dip on each butterflied breast.
3. Add 3 asparagus spears to each breast.
4. Fold the dip- and asparagus-filled chicken back into one whole breast and secure with cooking twine.
5. Season with salt and pepper and bake for 35 minutes.

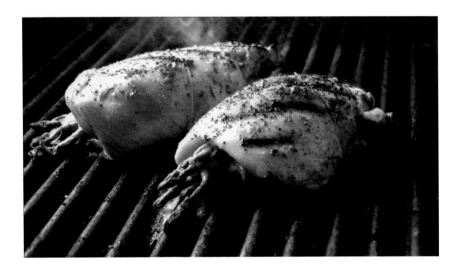

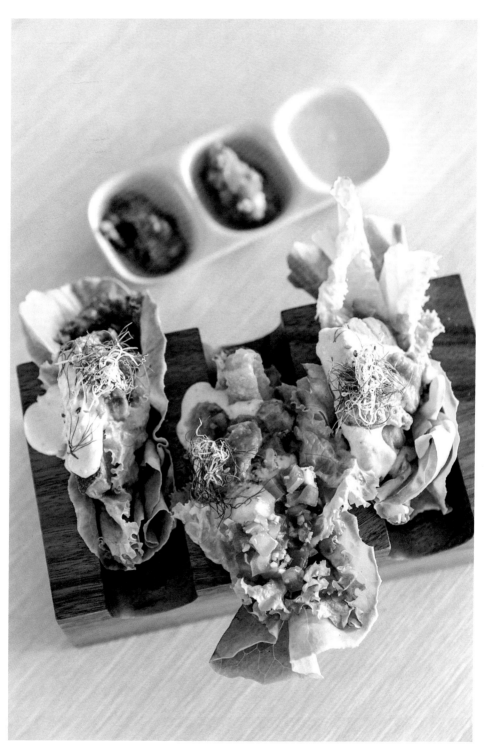

The Doctors Weight Loss Diet

Simple Salmon Taco Lettuce Wraps

This simple recipe is light and refreshing but filled with flavor. Reminiscent of traditional seaside Mexican cuisine, the healthy fats will keep you satisfied while the low-glycemic carbohydrates will provide antioxidants and fiber. Brighten these wraps up by squeezing fresh lime on top.

SERVES 2

1 tablespoon oil
1 pound salmon
Salt and pepper, to taste
1 head butter lettuce
1 avocado, mashed
2 tablespoons Greek
   yogurt
2 tablespoons pico de
   gallo or salsa
1 lemon, cut in half.

1. Heat the oil in a medium pan and add the salmon.
2. Add salt and pepper to taste, and cook over medium heat until cooked through. Break the salmon apart while cooking—leaving the skin on or removing is optional.
3. Display the lettuce, mashed avocado, Greek yogurt, salsa, and lemon.
4. Assemble the tacos by scooping the cooked salmon into individual lettuce cups and topping with your chosen add-ons and freshly squeezed lemon.

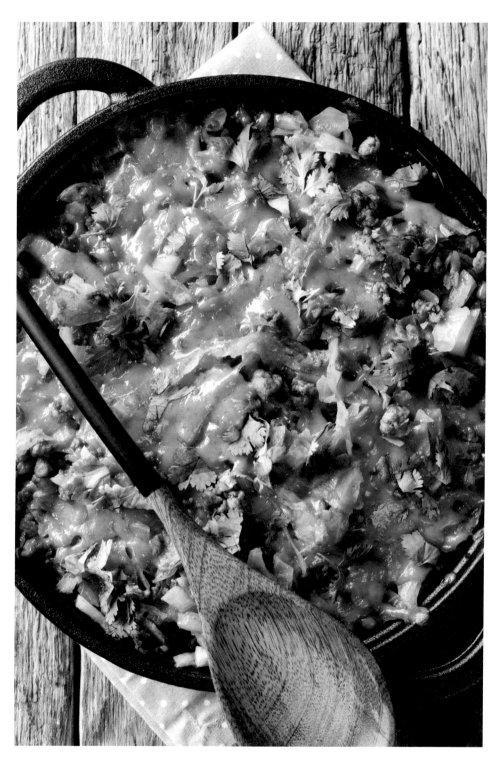

The Doctors Weight Loss Diet

Cheesy Beef Cabbage Roll Casserole

This is a casserole take on the classic cabbage roll dish, but it has some added cheese for a rich and creamy texture. To batch cook, simply double, triple, or even quadruple this recipe as this casserole is freezer-friendly. Serve warm with a small arugula salad.

SERVES 4–5

2 pounds ground beef

4 cups cabbage, shredded

½ yellow onion, thinly sliced

¾ cup sour cream

2 teaspoons garlic powder

Salt and pepper, to taste

1 cup shredded cheddar cheese, divided

Cilantro for garnish (optional)

1. Preheat the oven to 400°F.
2. In a large pan over medium-high heat, brown the ground beef, while breaking it into pieces with a spatula, for 3 to 4 minutes.
3. Add the cabbage and onion and combine; continue to cook for 5 to 6 minutes while stirring and breaking up the beef.
4. Remove from the heat and add the sour cream, stirring until combined. Add the garlic powder, salt, pepper, and half of the shredded cheddar cheese while mixing.
5. Pour into a baking dish and bake for 30 minutes. Top with the remainder of the shredded cheese and return to the oven until cheese is melted and browned, around 5 minutes. Garnish with cilantro (optional).

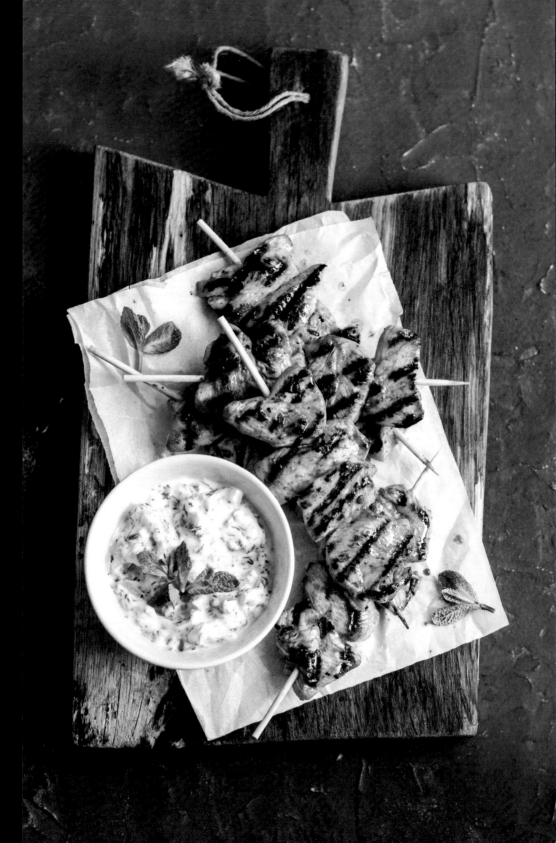

Spiced Chicken Skewers with Tahini-Yogurt Dip

This low-carb dish will satisfy your Indian food cravings without the use of any rice or legumes. If you're unfamiliar with the spice, garam masala is used in a variety of curry and lentil dishes and can be found in many mainstream grocery stores. If you're in a red-meat mood, simply replace the chicken with steak.

SERVES 3

1 cup plain Greek yogurt

¼ cup chopped fresh parsley

¼ cup tahini

2 tablespoons lemon juice

1 clove garlic

¾ teaspoon salt, divided

1 tablespoon oil

2 teaspoons garam masala

1 pound boneless, skinless chicken breasts, cut into 1-inch pieces

1. Prepare a grill with nonstick cooking spray for direct cooking, or preheat the broiler.
2. For the tahini-yogurt dip, combine the yogurt, parsley, tahini, lemon juice, garlic, and ¼ teaspoon salt in a food processor or blender; process until combined and set aside.
3. Combine the oil, garam masala, and remaining salt in a medium bowl. Add the chicken and toss to evenly coat. Thread the chicken on 8 (6-inch) metal or wooden skewers.
4. Grill the chicken skewers over medium-high heat or broil for 5 minutes per side or until the chicken is no longer pink. Serve with the tahini-yogurt dip.

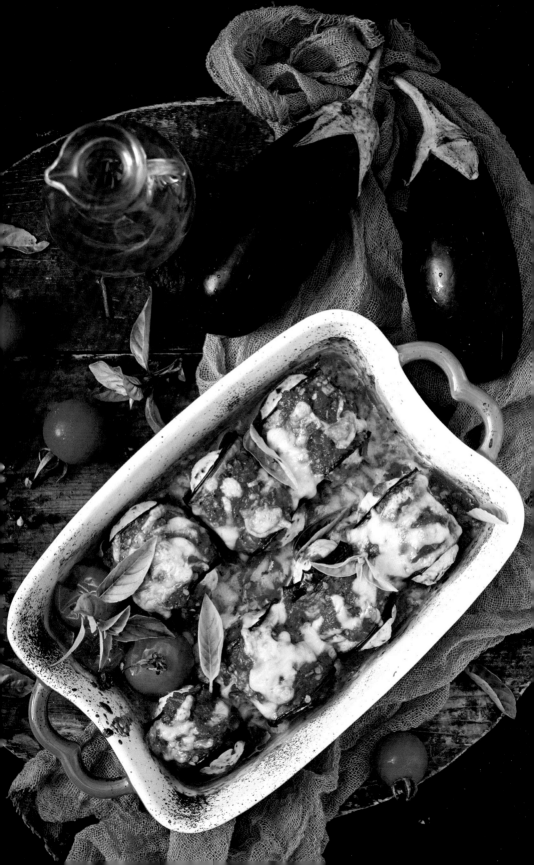

Italian Eggplant Roll-Ups

If you're craving lasagna, this low-carb dish has all of the elements but is far less labor-intensive. These roll-ups are just the base of endless opportunities—other ingredients such as spicy sausage and bell peppers make wonderful additions. Pair with a crisp Caesar salad for an Italian experience without the carbohydrates.

SERVES 6

1 large eggplant
1 cup cottage cheese or ricotta cheese
½ cup shredded mozzarella cheese
Salt and pepper, to taste
Garlic powder, to taste
1 teaspoon Italian seasoning mix
½ cup low-sugar marinara sauce

1. With the stem side up, stand the eggplant and cut it lengthwise into ¼-inch slices, for a total of around six portions.
2. Rub both sides of each eggplant slice with salt and pepper, to taste.
3. Place the eggplant slices on a layer of paper towels and allow them to "sweat" for 15 minutes.
4. Preheat the oven to 350°F.
5. Pat the eggplant dry with fresh paper towels and transfer the slices to a rimmed baking sheet.
6. Bake the eggplant until it is barely tender, about 15 minutes. Be sure not to overcook it.
7. While the eggplant slices are in the oven, place the cottage cheese, mozzarella, salt and pepper, garlic powder, and Italian seasoning in a medium bowl and combine. Set the bowl aside.
8. Remove the eggplant from the oven and allow them to cool for 5 minutes.
9. Raise the oven temperature to 400°F.
10. Spoon ¼ cup of the marinara sauce into the bottom of a 13x9-inch baking dish.
11. Spoon 2 tablespoons of the cottage cheese mixture onto an eggplant slice. Roll it up and place it, seam-side down, on the marinara sauce in the baking dish. Repeat until all slices have been filled, folded, and placed.
12. Top the roll-ups with the remaining marinara sauce and bake for 20 minutes.

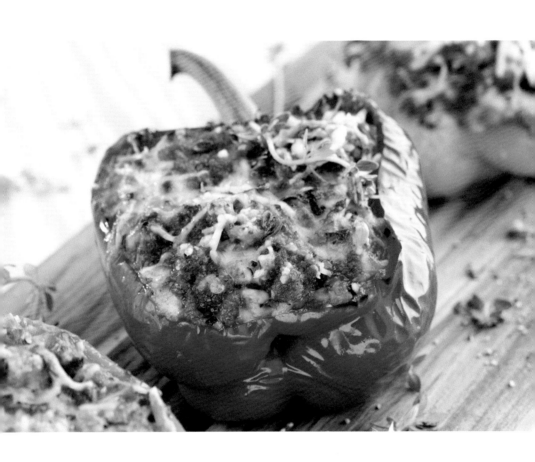

The Doctors Weight Loss Diet

Low-Carb Stuffed Peppers

Stuffed peppers are the quintessential comfort food and are still hearty without the addition of rice. This dish can be made in larger batches ahead of time and reheated for a meal on the go. Stuffed peppers are a complete dish on their own or can be paired with an arugula salad.

SERVES 2

1 cup riced cauliflower
1 tablespoon oil
1 teaspoon dried
    oregano, divided
Salt and pepper, to taste
6 ounces Italian sweet
    or hot sausage,
    casing removed
½ cup grated provolone
    cheese, divided
2 large red bell peppers

1. Preheat the oven to 350°F.
2. Place the cauliflower rice, oil, half the oregano, salt, and pepper in a large sauté pan over medium heat. Cover the pan to steam until tender, about 6 minutes. Remove the pan from the heat and set aside.
3. In another pan, cook the sausage (while breaking it apart), remaining oregano, salt, and pepper, until the sausage is no longer pink, around 8 minutes. Set the pan aside.
4. Add the sausage, the fat from the pan, and the cauliflower rice to a large bowl with ¼ cup of the cheese. Stir to combine and adjust seasonings if necessary, and set the bowl aside.
5. Cut the bell peppers lengthwise and remove the membranes. Place the peppers cut-side up in a baking dish and spoon the sausage mixture into each pepper half. Top with a sprinkle of cheese.
6. Cover the dish with foil and bake for 25 minutes. Remove the foil and bake for 10 more minutes, or until the cheese is bubbly.

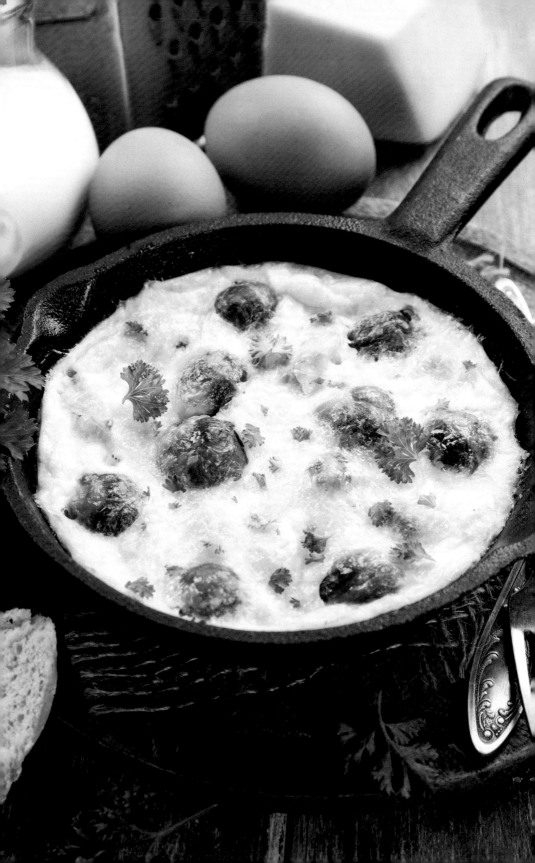

Creamy Brussels Skillet Casserole

Even if you don't like Brussels sprouts, you will love them this way. This creamy and cheesy dish stands up on its own, or you can use this recipe as a base, adding chicken or salmon. This casserole can be prepared ahead of time as it keeps well in the refrigerator and can be easily reheated.

SERVES 4

8 slices bacon, chopped
2 pounds Brussels
    sprouts, trimmed and
    halved
2 garlic cloves, minced
1½ cups heavy cream
1 tablespoon lemon
    juice
½ cup shredded
    Parmesan cheese
Salt and pepper, to taste

1. Place a large deep skillet over medium heat. Add the bacon and cook until browned. Remove the bacon and set aside, keeping the bacon fat in the pan.
2. Add the Brussels sprouts and cover the pan. Cook until tender, stirring occasionally, around 8 to 9 minutes.
3. Add the garlic and stir for 1 minute until fragrant. Add the cream and bring to a simmer.
4. Stir in the lemon juice and then sprinkle with the Parmesan cheese, and stir to combine.
5. Season with salt and pepper, bring to a simmer, and then remove from the heat. Garnish with the reserved bacon.

Au Gratin Radishes

Your favorite potatoes au gratin can be re-created in the low-carb way by replacing potatoes with radishes. Radishes are extremely low in carbo-hydrates but can mimic the potato texture especially when prepared in a creamy cheese sauce. This recipe serves as an excellent base, but you can use any additions you like such as cooked chicken, ground beef, or bacon.

SERVES 4–6

3 tablespoons butter
½ large yellow onion, finely chopped
1 cup heavy whipping cream
⅓ cup Parmesan cheese, shredded
1 cup cheddar cheese, shredded
Salt and pepper, to taste
5 cups sliced radishes
Chopped scallions for garnish

1. Preheat the oven to 350°F.
2. In a medium pot, melt the butter over low heat.
3. Add the onion and let cook until slightly tender, around 3 minutes.
4. Add the heavy whipping cream and let simmer for 4 to 5 more minutes, stirring occasionally.
5. Slowly add all of the cheese, stirring as you slowly add, to melt into a smooth, creamy mixture.
6. Add the salt and pepper to taste and stir.
7. Remove from the heat, and grease an 8- or 9-inch square baking pan.
8. Layer with radishes to cover the bottom. If you are using additional ingredients like bacon or cooked chicken, add them on top of the radishes. Add some of the melted cheese mixture.
9. Repeat step 8 until you are out of radishes and melted cheese, and bake for 1 hour.

Bun-less Philly Cheesesteaks

The flavor in a good Philly cheesesteak lies in the steak, onions, peppers, and melting provolone, so you definitely won't miss the bun in this dish. This recipe is only a base. It will work with several variations of produce and cheese, so be sure to experiment!

SERVES 2

1 tablespoon butter
1 cup white mushrooms
½ cup chopped onions
⅓ cup chopped green
   bell pepper
½ teaspoon garlic
   powder
8 ounces rare roast beef
   slices
2 slices provolone
   cheese
Salt and pepper, to taste

1. In a medium pan over medium heat, melt the butter and then add the mushrooms, onions, bell pepper, and garlic powder. Cook until the produce is soft, about 4 to 5 minutes.
2. Slice the roast beef into strips or 1-inch squares.
3. Add the roast beef to the pan and toss with the produce mixture for 1 minute, until heated through.
4. Reduce the heat to low and top the roast beef mixture with the provolone cheese. Cover the pan with a lid and continue to heat for 2 to 3 minutes, until the cheese is melted. Season with salt and pepper, to taste.

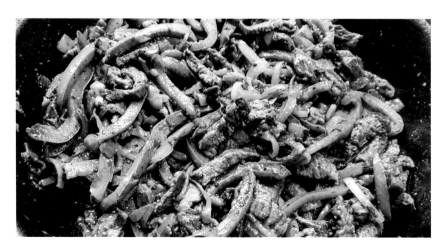

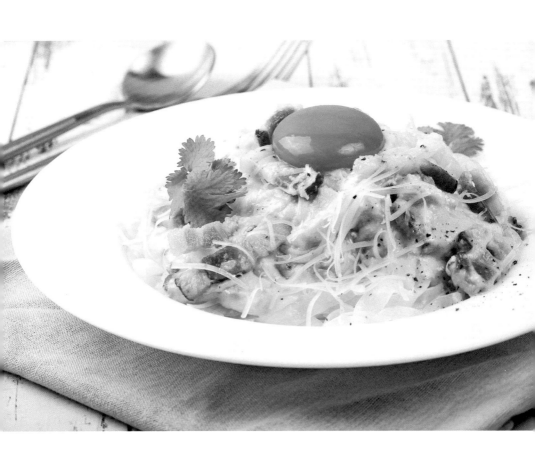

The Doctors Weight Loss Diet

Shirataki Carbonara

This rendition is a revised take on the old classic. Even if your family isn't following the same low-carb plan, they will be sure to love this rich and creamy pasta dish. If you can't find shirataki noodles at your local grocery store, zoodles (zucchini noodles) work well as a substitution.

SERVES 2

4 slices bacon

3 ounces chicken breast, chopped

1 (7-ounce) packet shirataki noodles

1 large egg yolk

2–3 tablespoons Parmesan cheese

1 cup heavy cream

1. Dice the bacon and cook over medium heat until it changes color but does not get crispy. Remove from the pan and set aside.

2. Cook the chopped chicken pieces over medium heat in the same pan as the bacon, until almost fully cooked, around 6 minutes. Remove the chicken and set aside.

3. Meanwhile, dry fry (using a dry frying pan with no oil or butter) the shirataki noodles so that all excess water evaporates, around 7 minutes.

4. In a small bowl, thoroughly combine the egg yolk and Parmesan cheese until you have a smooth paste.

5. In the same pan used for the bacon and chicken, add half of the cream and add the Parmesan-egg mixture and combine over medium heat. This may take a few minutes until it is smooth.

6. Add the remaining cream, chicken, and bacon and incorporate.

7. Combine the chicken and bacon sauce with the noodles and serve hot.

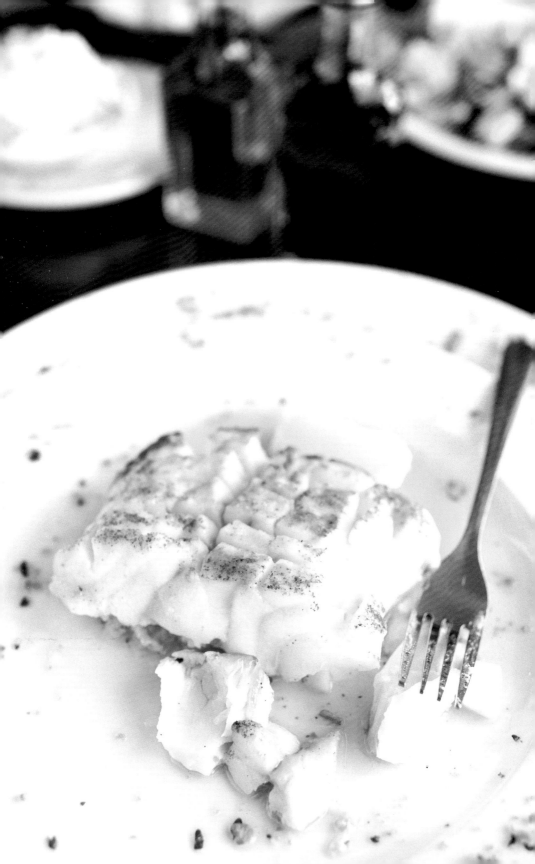

Easy Bake Lemon Butter Fish

If you are newer to seafood, this is a wonderful recipe to try as it has a very mild fish taste—if you like chicken, you will probably enjoy this dish! Mild whitefish pairs well with steamed or sautéed green beans, with a generous amount of freshly squeezed lemon on top. To brighten it up even more, add some more fresh herbs in addition to the parsley.

SERVES 4

¼ cup melted butter
4 garlic cloves, minced
Zest and juice of
    1 lemon, plus 1 lemon,
    sliced
2 tablespoons fresh
    parsley, minced
Salt and pepper, to taste
4 fillets of cod, halibut,
    or rockfish

1. Preheat the oven to 425°F.
2. In a bowl, combine the butter, garlic, lemon zest, lemon juice, and parsley; season with salt and pepper to taste.
3. Place the fish in a greased baking dish.
4. Pour the lemon butter mixture over the fish and top with fresh lemon slices.
5. Bake for 12 to 15 minutes, or until fish is flaky and cooked through.
6. Serve the fish topped with fresh parsley and freshly squeezed lemon juice.

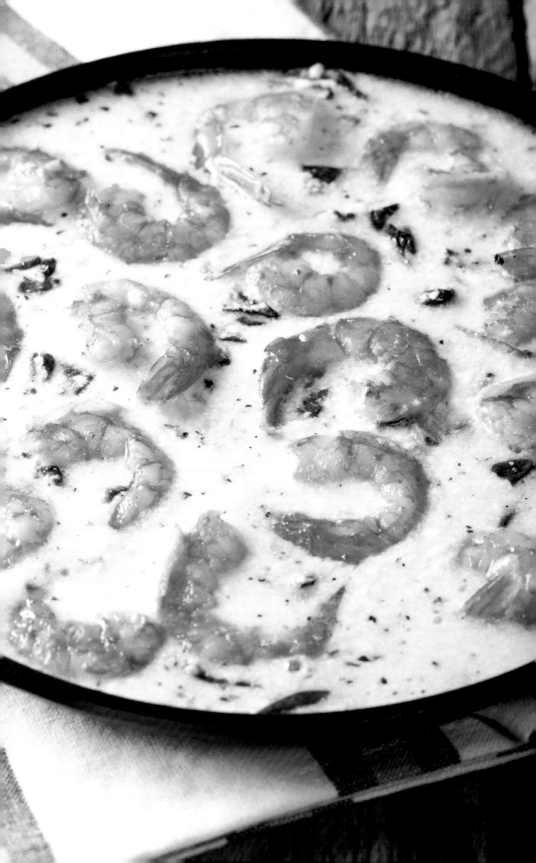

Creamy Tuscan Shrimp

If you're not a fan of shellfish, this recipe works just as well with chicken. This dish pairs well with a crisp salad or can be served over riced cauliflower for an even heartier meal.

SERVES 3–4

2 tablespoons olive oil

2 tablespoons butter

1 pound shrimp, deveined, and tails removed

Salt and pepper, to taste

3–4 cloves garlic, minced

1 cup halved cherry or grape tomatoes

3–4 cups baby spinach

¾ cup heavy cream

¼ cup freshly grated Parmesan

2 tablespoons basil, thinly sliced

1. Heat the oil and butter in a large skillet over medium-high heat, until the oil is very hot and the butter has melted.
2. Carefully add the shrimp and sprinkle with salt and pepper; sauté for 1 minute on each side.
3. Remove the shrimp from the pan and set aside. Add the garlic, tomatoes, and spinach to the same pan. Sauté until the garlic is fragrant, about 1 minute.
4. Stir in the cream, Parmesan cheese, and basil, and reduce the heat to medium. Simmer until the sauce is slightly reduced, about 2 to 3 minutes.
5. Return the shrimp to the pan and stir to combine. Serve warm.

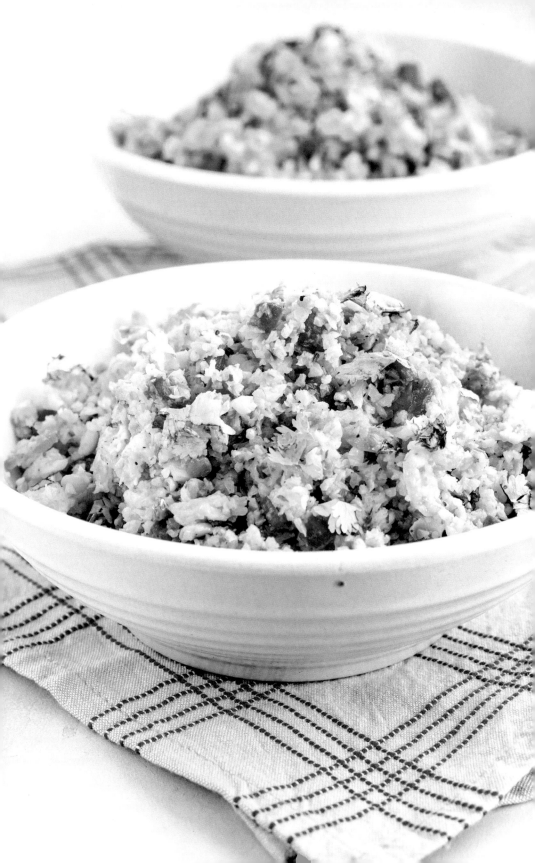

Cauliflower Fried Rice

If you're in the mood for Chinese food, this recipe will still keep your macros in line to get results. You can add any protein you choose to make it a complete meal or feel free to have it on its own. Chicken, shrimp, or chunks of salmon are complementary additions to this dish.

SERVES 4

3 eggs
1 tablespoon coconut oil
1 tablespoon sesame oil
½ small onion, diced fine
5 scallions, diced
½ cup red bell pepper, diced
2 garlic cloves, minced
20 ounces riced cauliflower (store-bought is okay)
3 tablespoons soy sauce, or more to taste
1 teaspoon ginger powder
1 tablespoon coconut aminos

1. Beat the eggs in a small bowl with a fork.
2. Heat a large sauté pan or wok over medium heat and add the coconut oil. Add the eggs and cook, turning a few times until set, then set aside on a plate.
3. In the same pan, add the sesame oil and sauté the onion, scallions, bell pepper, and garlic for about 4 to 5 minutes, or until soft. Raise the heat to medium-high.
4. Add the riced cauliflower to the pan along with the soy sauce, ginger, and the coconut aminos. Mix, cover, and cook for 5 to 6 minutes, stirring frequently, until the cauliflower is slightly crispy on the outside but tender on the inside.
5. Add the scrambled eggs and combine, then remove from the heat to serve.

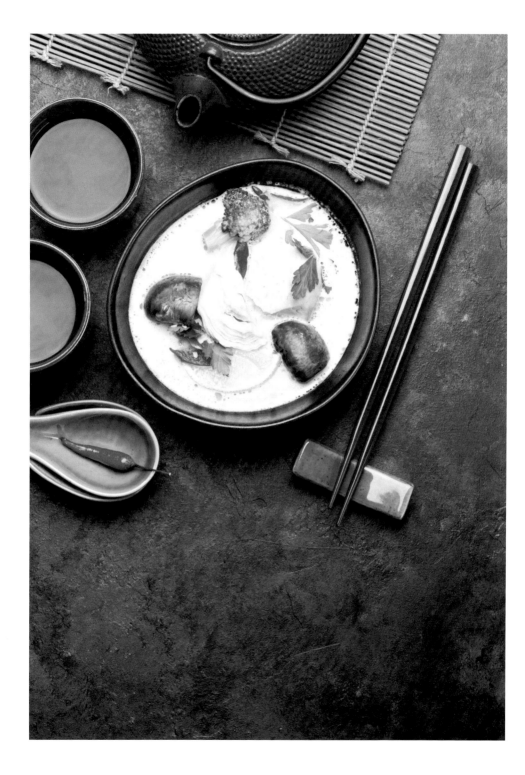

The Doctors Weight Loss Diet

Tom Kha Thai Soup

Although this is just a soup, it's aromatic, silky, and a complete meal in one go, with lots of filling ingredients. If you're looking for a completely different chicken and broccoli dish, this one is sure to do the trick.

SERVES 4–6

2 cups broccoli florets, chopped into bite-size pieces

2 stalks fresh lemongrass, tough outer layers removed

1-inch piece ginger, peeled

1 tablespoon lime zest

¼ cup lime juice

6 cups low-sodium chicken broth

1½ pounds boneless, skinless chicken thighs, cut into 1-inch pieces

8 ounces shiitake or oyster mushrooms, stemmed and cut into bite-size pieces

1 (13.5-ounce) can coconut milk

2 tablespoons fish sauce

1 tablespoon coconut aminos

Cilantro leaves, lime wedges, and thinly sliced red jalapeño pepper, for serving (optional)

1. Over high heat, steam the broccoli until slightly tender, around 12 minutes.
2. Meanwhile, using the back of a knife, lightly smash the lemongrass and ginger; cut the lemongrass into four-inch pieces.
3. Bring the lemongrass, ginger, lime zest, lime juice, and broth to a boil in a large saucepan. Reduce the heat and simmer until flavors are melded, around 8 to 10 minutes.
4. Strain the broth into a clean saucepan; discard the solids.
5. Add the chicken and return to a boil. Reduce the heat, add the mushrooms, and simmer, stirring occasionally, until the chicken is cooked through and the mushrooms are soft, around 20 to 25 minutes.
6. Mix in the coconut milk, fish sauce, and coconut aminos.
7. Serve with the cilantro leaves, lime wedges, and jalapeño pepper (optional).

Mediterranean Chicken Pesto Casserole

Between the Mediterranean superstars, the olives, feta cheese, and pesto pack this creamy chicken dish with flavor, and it's simple to make. A crisp side salad makes the perfect pairing to this comfort food dish.

SERVES 4

1½ pounds chicken breasts or boneless chicken thighs
Salt and pepper, to taste
2 tablespoons butter or ghee
5 tablespoons pesto (page 261, or store-bought)
1¼ cups heavy cream
3 ounces pitted olives
5 ounces feta cheese, diced
1 garlic clove, minced
Fresh parsley for garnish

1. Preheat the oven to 400°F.
2. Cut the chicken into bite-size pieces and season with salt and pepper.
3. Add the butter to a large skillet and cook over medium-high heat, until browned on all sides, but not cooked all of the way through.
4. Mix the pesto and cream in a bowl.
5. Place the chicken, olives, feta cheese, and garlic in a baking dish. Add the pesto/cream mixture.
6. Bake in the oven until the dish turns bubbly and light brown around the edges, around 25 minutes.
7. Garnish with parsley and serve.

CHAPTER 22

Doctors Weight Loss Soups, Sides, and Sauces

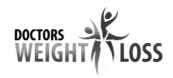

Broccoli and Cheese Soup

SERVES 4–6

1 tablespoon oil
4 cloves garlic,
   minced
3½ cups chicken
   broth (or vegetable
   or bone broth)
1 cup heavy cream
4 cups broccoli,
   chopped into
   small florets
3 cups cheddar
   cheese

1. In a large pot over medium heat, add the oil and sauté the garlic until fragrant, about 1 minute.
2. Add the chicken broth, cream, and chopped broccoli. Increase the heat to bring to a boil.
3. Once it begins to boil, reduce the heat and simmer for 15 to 20 minutes, until the broccoli is tender.
4. Add ½ cup of the cheddar cheese, simmer, and stir until melted. Repeat this process ½ cup at a time until all the cheese is used. Be sure to keep the heat at a very low simmer and avoid high heat, to prevent seizing.
5. Remove from the heat immediately once all the cheese melts, and serve.

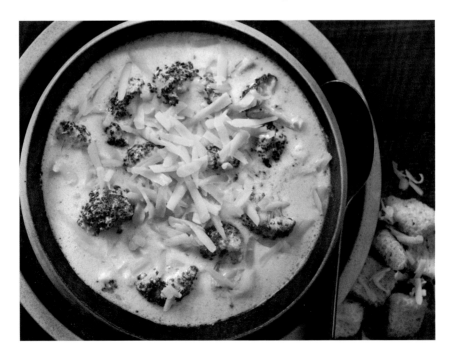

Taco Soup

SERVES 4–6

1 pound ground beef

3 tablespoons low-sugar taco seasoning, divided

4 cups beef bone broth (or any broth of choice), divided

2 (14.5-ounce) cans diced tomatoes (with liquid)

¾ cup ranch dressing

1. Brown the ground beef in a large pot over medium-high heat for 7 to 10 minutes, or until no longer pink. Drain if desired.
2. Add 2 tablespoons of the taco seasoning and ¾ cup of the broth. Simmer for 4 to 5 minutes, or until the liquid is mostly gone.
3. Add the remaining broth, diced tomatoes (with liquid), and the remaining tablespoon of taco seasoning, and combine.
4. Bring to a low boil and simmer for 8 to 10 minutes, and remove from the heat.
5. Wait 2 minutes and then stir in the ranch dressing. Add any desired garnishes such as sour cream, scallions, cheddar cheese, cilantro, or avocado.

Creamy Spinach Soup

SERVES 4–6

3 cups raw spinach
3 garlic cloves, minced
2 tablespoons butter or ghee
1½ cups bone broth or vegetable broth
1 cup heavy cream
1 cup shredded mozzarella cheese (optional)

1. Over medium heat in a large pan, sauté the spinach and garlic in butter until the spinach is wilted, around 5 minutes.
2. Add the bone broth and cream and combine.
3. Transfer to a blender and blend for 2 to 3 minutes.
4. Transfer back to the pan until the soup boils.
5. Add the mozzarella cheese and stir until melted (optional).

Cream of Mushroom Soup

SERVES 4–5

1 tablespoon oil
½ large onion, diced
2½ cups mushrooms, sliced
6 cloves garlic, minced
2 cups chicken or vegetable broth
1 cup heavy cream
1 cup unsweetened almond milk
Salt and pepper, to taste

1. In a large pot over medium heat, sauté the onions and mushrooms in oil for about 10 to 15 minutes, stirring occasionally, until lightly browned. Add the garlic and cook for 2 more minutes.
2. Add the chicken broth, cream, almond milk, salt, and pepper. Bring to a boil, then simmer for 15 minutes, stirring occasionally.
3. Use an immersion blender to puree until smooth, or puree in batches in a regular blender.

Bone Broth

SERVES 4

1 gallon water

2 tablespoons apple cider vinegar

2–4 pounds beef or poultry bones

Salt and pepper, to taste

1. Place all the ingredients in a large pot or slow cooker and bring to a boil.
2. Reduce to a low simmer and cook for 12 to 24 hours. The longer it cooks, the better it will taste and more nutritious it will be.
3. Allow the broth to cool. Strain it into a large container and discard the solids.

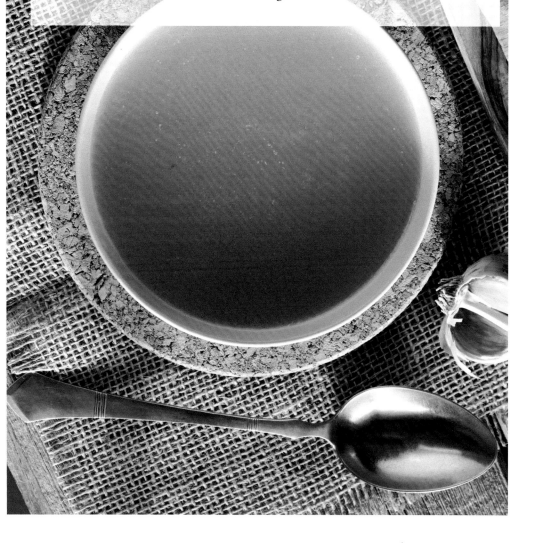

Chicken Vegetable Soup

SERVES 4

2 tablespoons oil

1 medium onion, chopped

5 cloves garlic, smashed

3 cups riced cauliflower

¾ teaspoon crushed red pepper flakes

4 stalks celery, thinly sliced

6 cups low-sodium chicken broth or bone broth

2 boneless, skinless chicken breasts

Salt and pepper, to taste

1. In a large pot over medium heat, heat the oil and add the onion and garlic, cooking until they begin to brown.
2. Add the riced cauliflower to the pot and cook over medium-high heat until it begins to brown, about 8 minutes.
3. Add the red pepper flakes, celery, and chicken broth and bring to a simmer.
4. Add the chicken breasts and let cook slowly until they reach an internal temperature of 165°F, about 15 minutes. Remove the chicken from the pot and shred once it is cool enough to handle. Meanwhile, continue simmering until vegetables are tender, 3 to 5 minutes more.
5. Add the shredded chicken back to the soup and season to taste with salt and pepper.

Jalapeño Poppers

SERVES 3

5 slices bacon

6 jalapeño peppers

3 ounces cream cheese, softened

¼ cup shredded cheddar cheese

½ teaspoon garlic powder

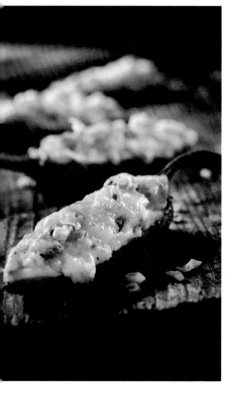

1. Preheat the oven to 400°F.
2. In pan over medium heat, cook the bacon until crispy, around 10 minutes, flipping over occasionally. Chop and set aside.
3. Meanwhile, line a baking sheet with parchment paper.
4. Slice the jalapeños in half lengthwise, and remove the inner seeds and membranes.
5. In a medium bowl, combine the cream cheese, cheddar cheese, garlic powder, and cooked bacon.
6. Spoon the cheese mixture into each jalapeño half and set the filled peppers cheese-side up on the lined baking sheet.
7. Bake for 18 to 20 minutes until the cheese is melted and slightly crisp on top.

Cauliflower Hummus

SERVES 4

1 medium head
  cauliflower
4 tablespoons extra-
  virgin olive oil
½ cup tahini
2 garlic cloves
⅓ cup lemon juice
1 teaspoon salt
½ teaspoon ground
  black pepper
Chopped fresh parsley,
  to taste (optional)

1. Preheat the oven to 375°F and chop the
   cauliflower into small florets.
2. Toss cauliflower in extra-virgin olive oil
   and place on a baking sheet; roast until
   tender, about 20 minutes.
3. Place the roasted cauliflower in a food
   processor or blender and combine with
   all other ingredients.

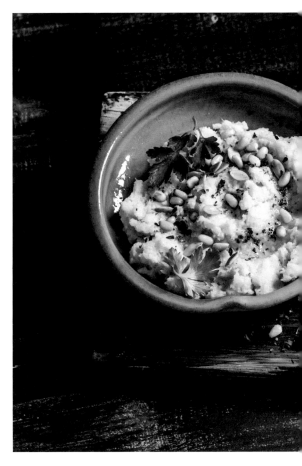

Spinach Artichoke Dip

MAKES 2 CUPS

1 (9-ounce) box frozen
spinach, defrosted
14 ounces canned
artichoke hearts
8 ounces cream cheese
¼ cup sour cream
1 teaspoon garlic
powder
Salt and pepper, to taste
½ teaspoon red pepper
flakes (optional)
1 cup mozzarella

1. Place the defrosted spinach and artichokes in a colander and press firmly to extract as much liquid as possible, and set aside.
2. Add the cream cheese to a medium microwave-safe bowl and soften in the microwave for 30 seconds or until the cream cheese is the same consistency as mayonnaise.
3. Add the spinach, artichokes, sour cream, garlic powder, salt and pepper, and red pepper flakes (optional) and combine.
4. Fold in the mozzarella cheese.
5. Refrigerate for at least 1 hour and serve with vegetables to dip or as a steak topper or baked salmon or chicken stuffer.

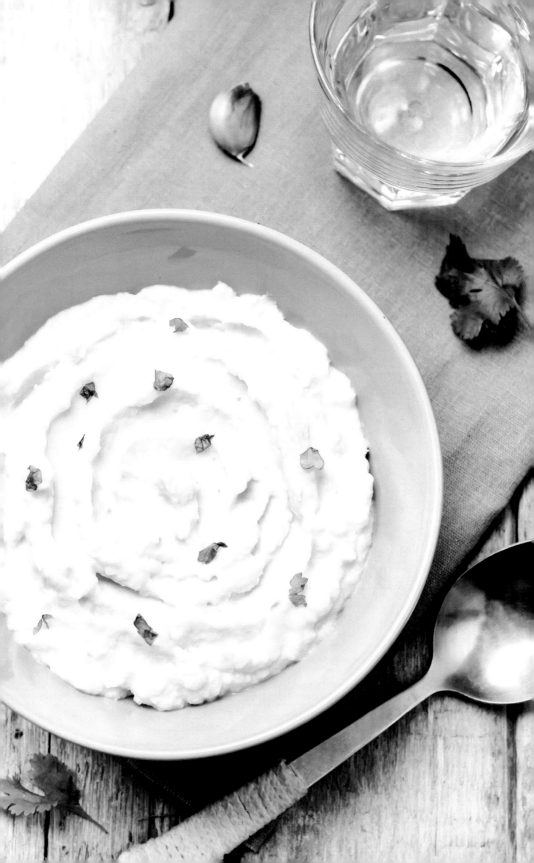

Four-Ingredient Salmon Dip

MAKES 2 CUPS

8 ounces smoked
  salmon, finely
  chopped
8 ounces crème fraîche
Juice from 2 lemons
1–2 tablespoons fresh
  dill, finely chopped

1. In a medium bowl, combine the salmon
   and crème fraîche until the crème fraîche
   turns pink.
2. Add the lemon juice and dill and mix
   until thoroughly incorporated.
3. Serve with endive leaves or radish slices
   to dip.

Mashed Cauliflower

SERVES 4

1 head cauliflower
½ cup grated Parmesan
  cheese

1. Chop the cauliflower and steam until
   extremely tender.
2. Using a potato masher or fork, mash into
   a mashed potato-like texture.
3. Add grated Parmesan and thoroughly
   combine.

Asparagus in Gorgonzola Sauce

SERVES 2

10 asparagus spears
Gorgonzola sauce
  (page 254)

1. Steam the asparagus spears until tender,
   around 10 minutes.
2. Top with the Gorgonzola sauce.

Parmesan Roasted Fennel

SERVES 2

1 large fennel bulb,
    quartered, and stems
    removed
2 tablespoons grated
    Parmesan cheese
1 tablespoon extra-
    virgin olive oil

1. Boil or steam the quartered fennel until
   tender; toss in extra-virgin olive oil.
2. Roast for 10 minutes at 400°F; sprinkle
   with Parmesan cheese and roast for
   2 additional minutes.

Creamy Cucumber Salad

SERVES 2

½ cup plain almond or
    coconut yogurt
1 scallion, chopped
1 tablespoon sliced red
    onion
Black pepper, to taste
1 tablespoon fresh
    dill, chopped, or
    ½ teaspoon dried dill
1 garlic clove, minced
½ cup cucumber, thinly
    sliced

1. Combine the yogurt with the scallion,
   red onion, pepper, dill, and garlic.
2. Add the cucumbers and toss until evenly
   coated.

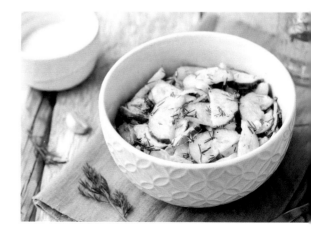

Zucchini Chips

SERVES 4

2 medium zucchini
1 tablespoon oil
Salt, to taste
Your favorite
    seasonings, to taste
    (optional)

1. Preheat the oven to 200°F and line two baking sheets with parchment paper.
2. Slice the zucchini into ⅛-inch slices (a mandoline works well).
3. Toss the zucchini slices in the oil, salt, and your favorite seasonings.
4. Place the slices side by side (they can touch but not overlap) and bake for about 2½ hours, rotating the pans halfway through.
5. The chips are done when they are golden and just starting to get crispy. Allow them to cool in the oven with the heat off and the door propped slightly open.

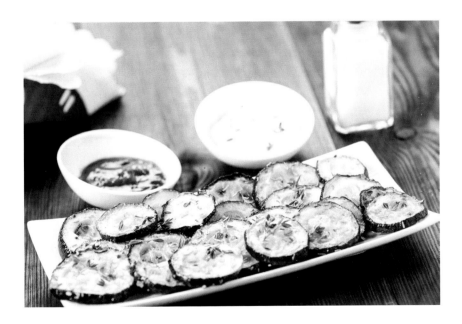

Creamy Alfredo Sauce

SERVES 4

⅓ cup butter
2 cloves garlic, pressed
4 ounces cream cheese,
  cubed
1 cup half-and-half
½ cup grated Parmesan
  cheese
½ teaspoon dried
  oregano
½ teaspoon salt
½ teaspoon black pepper

1. In a medium saucepan, melt the butter over medium heat. Add the garlic and thoroughly combine.
2. Add the cream cheese and whisk constantly until the cheese is melted. Slowly pour in the half-and-half and whisk continuously until smooth.
3. Gradually add the grated Parmesan, while whisking until combined.
4. Add the oregano, salt, and pepper and stir. Continue to simmer for 1 to 2 minutes, but do not let the sauce boil. Add more salt and pepper, to taste, if desired.
5. Remove from the heat and serve, or refrigerate in airtight containers for up to 5 days.

Ranch Dressing

MAKES 2 CUPS

1 cup mayonnaise
½ cup sour cream
2 teaspoons lemon juice
1 teaspoon dried dill
1 teaspoon dried chives
½ teaspoon garlic powder
½ teaspoon salt
½ teaspoon black pepper
¼ cup unsweetened almond
  milk

1. Whisk all the ingredients (except the almond milk) until thoroughly combined.
2. Gradually whisk in the almond milk until the desired consistency has been reached.
3. Refrigerate for at least 1 hour and up to 10 days.

Tzatziki

MAKES 1½ CUPS

1 cup Greek whole milk
   yogurt
1 small cucumber, diced
2 cloves garlic, minced
2 tablespoons fresh
   lemon juice
2 tablespoons fresh dill,
   chopped
1 tablespoon fresh mint,
   finely chopped
Salt and pepper to taste
   (optional)

1. In a medium mixing bowl, combine all
   the ingredients.
2. Store in an airtight container and
   refrigerate for up to 7 days.

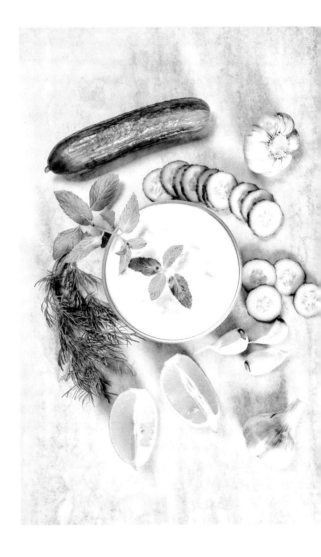

Picnic Salad Dressing

MAKES 1 CUP

⅔ cup mayonnaise
3 tablespoons apple
    cider vinegar
1 tablespoon Dijon
    mustard
Salt and pepper, to taste

1. In a medium bowl, combine all the ingredients.
2. Optionally, this dressing is great tossed with broccoli florets and diced onion, sunflower seeds, cooked bacon bits, and grated cheddar cheese for an easy broccoli salad.

Gorgonzola Sauce

MAKES 1 CUP

1 clove garlic, minced
2 tablespoons butter
⅓ cup crumbled
    Gorgonzola cheese
¼ cup grated Parmesan
    cheese
¼ cup heavy cream
1 teaspoon onion
    powder
Salt and pepper, to taste

1. In a small saucepan over low heat, combine the garlic and butter.
2. When the butter is melted, add the remaining ingredients, stir, and raise the heat to medium-high.
3. Allow the sauce to come to a simmer and continue to stir for 3 to 5 minutes, allowing it to reduce until the desired consistency is achieved.

Avocado Oil Mayonnaise

MAKES 1¼ CUPS

1 large egg, at room
   temperature
1 teaspoon Dijon
   mustard
2 teaspoons apple cider
   vinegar
¼ teaspoon salt
1 cup avocado oil

1. Crack the egg in a medium bowl and
   place all the other ingredients on top.
2. Using an immersion blender, blend on
   medium-high heat until a mayonnaise
   texture forms.
3. Place in an airtight container and store
   in the refrigerator for up to 2 weeks.

Dairy-Free Cashew Cheese Sauce

MAKES 2 CUPS

1½ cups raw cashew
   pieces
¼ cup nutritional yeast
   flakes
1 teaspoon salt
¼ teaspoon garlic
   powder
¾ cup water
3 tablespoons freshly
   squeezed lemon

1. In a food processor or blender, process
   the cashews into a fine powder, adding a
   drizzle of water if needed.
2. Add the nutritional yeast, salt, and garlic
   powder and process to combine.
3. Add the lemon juice and water and
   process until smooth.

Easy Caesar Dressing

MAKES 1½ CUPS

¾ cup mayonnaise
⅓ cup grated Parmesan
   cheese
2 cloves garlic, pressed
1 teaspoon anchovy
   paste
1 teaspoon lemon juice
½ teaspoon Dijon
   mustard
Salt and pepper, to taste

1. Place all the ingredients in a medium
   bowl and thoroughly combine.
2. Serve immediately or store in an airtight
   container in the refrigerator for up to
   1 week.

White Wine Sauce

MAKES 1 CUP

½ cup chicken broth
¼ cup white wine
Juice of ½ lemon
1 tablespoon minced
   shallot
1 clove garlic, minced
1 tablespoon butter
1 tablespoon extra-
   virgin olive oil
Black pepper, to taste

1. Combine all the ingredients in a pan and
   use as a simmer sauce.

Lemon Vinaigrette

MAKES 1 CUP

¼ cup red wine vinegar

2 tablespoons Dijon mustard

1 clove garlic, minced

1 teaspoon dried oregano

¼ teaspoon ground black pepper

½ cup olive oil

2 tablespoons fresh lemon juice

1. Whisk the vinegar, mustard, garlic, oregano, and black pepper in a small bowl until blended.
2. Drizzle in the oil, whisking until blended.
3. Beat the lemon juice into the mixture.

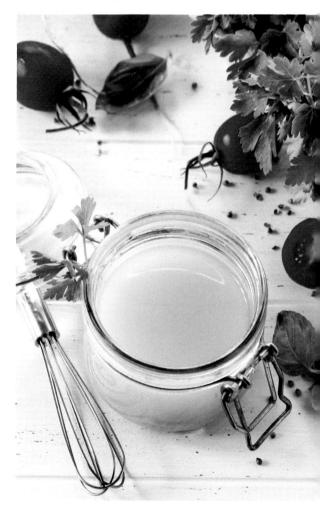

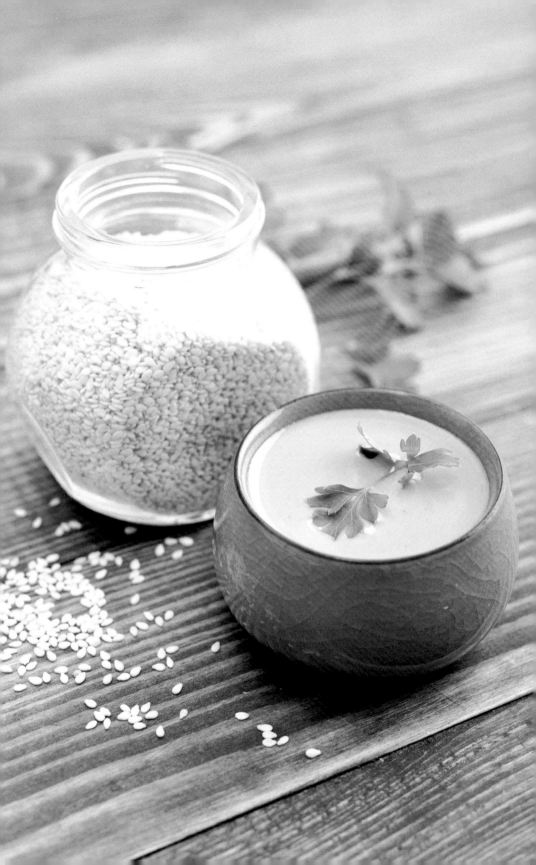

Creamy Tahini-Lemon Dressing

MAKES 1½ CUPS

½ cup tahini
2 cloves garlic, minced
4 tablespoons fresh
  lemon juice
1 tablespoon extra-
  virgin olive oil
⅓ cup water
Salt and pepper, to taste

1. Thoroughly combine all the ingredients;
   add more water if needed until the
   desired consistency is reached.
2. Store in the refrigerator in an airtight
   container for up to 7 days.

Smooth Tomato and Goat Cheese

MAKES 1 CUP

¼ cup crumbled goat
  cheese
2 tablespoons white
  wine vinegar
¼ cup extra-virgin olive
  oil
2 plum tomatoes,
  seeded and chopped
½ teaspoon salt
Freshly ground pepper,
  to taste
1 tablespoon chopped
  fresh tarragon
  (optional)

1. Blend all the ingredients together until
   the mixture is creamy and smooth (can
   be refrigerated for up to 3 days).

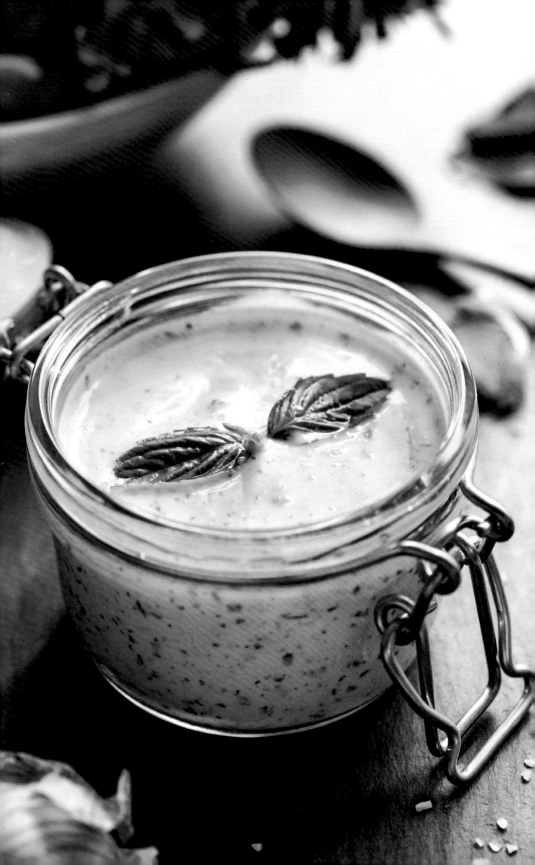

Creamy Cucumber Vinaigrette

MAKES 1 CUP

1 small cucumber, peeled,
    seeded, and chopped
¼ cup extra-virgin olive oil
2 tablespoons red wine
    vinegar
2 tablespoons chopped fresh
    chives
2 tablespoons chopped fresh
    parsley
2 tablespoons Greek yogurt
1 teaspoon prepared
    horseradish (optional)

1. Blend all the ingredients together until the mixture is creamy and smooth.

Green Pesto

MAKES 2 CUPS

1½ cups fresh basil leaves
    (packed)
¼ teaspoon freshly ground
    black pepper
¼ cup freshly grated
    Parmigiano-Reggiano
    (optional)
2 tablespoons pine nuts or
    walnuts
1 teaspoon minced garlic
½ cup extra-virgin olive oil

1. Using a food processor or blender, combine the basil and pepper and process/blend for a few seconds until the basil is chopped.
2. Add the cheese, pine nuts, and garlic and, while the processor is running, add the oil in a thin, steady stream until you have reached a smooth consistency.

Horseradish Cream Sauce

MAKES 1½ CUPS

1 cup Greek yogurt
¼ cup grated fresh
    horseradish
1 tablespoon Dijon
    mustard
1 teaspoon white wine
    vinegar
¼ teaspoon freshly
    ground black pepper

1. Place all of the ingredients into a medium mixing bowl and whisk until the mixture is smooth and creamy.
2. Refrigerate for at least 4 hours to allow flavors to meld.

Chimichurri Sauce

MAKES 1 CUP

1 bunch parsley, finely
    chopped
1 bunch cilantro, finely
    chopped
3 tablespoons capers,
    finely chopped
2 garlic cloves, minced
1½ tablespoons red wine
    vinegar
½ teaspoon red pepper
    flakes
½ teaspoon ground
    black pepper
½ cup extra-virgin olive
    oil

1. Put the parsley, cilantro, capers, and garlic in a medium mixing bowl and toss to combine.
2. Add the vinegar, red pepper, and black pepper, and stir.
3. Pour in the olive oil and mix until well combined; let sit for 30 minutes so that the flavors blend.

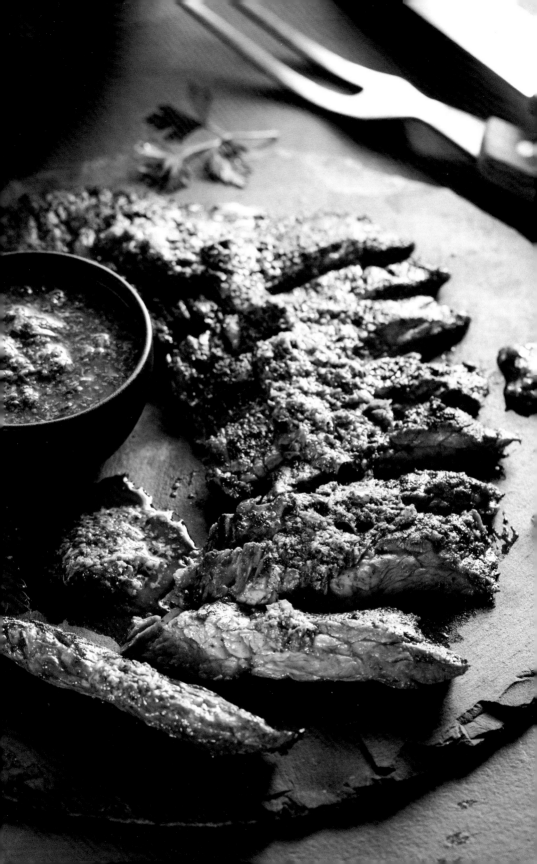

References

Avena, N., P. Rada, and B. Hoebel. "Evidence for Sugar Addiction: Behavioral and Neurochemical Effects of Intermittent, Excessive Sugar Intake." NCBI. *Neuroscience and Biobehavioral Reviews*, January 2008. https://www.ncbi.nlm.nih.gov/pmc/articles/PMC2235907/.

Calder, P. C.; "Marine Omega-3 Fatty Acids and Inflammatory Processes: Effects, Mechanisms and Clinical Relevance," NCBI. April 2015, https://pubmed.ncbi.nlm.nih.gov/25149823/.

Callegaro, D., and J. Tirapegui. "[Comparison of the Nutritional Value between Brown Rice and White Rice]." NCBI. October/November 1996. Accessed April 14, 2019. https://www.ncbi.nlm.nih.gov/pubmed/9302338.

Chinwong, S., D. Chinwong, and A. Mangklabruks. "Daily Consumption of Virgin Coconut Oil Increases High-Density Lipoprotein Cholesterol Levels in Healthy Volunteers: A Randomized Crossover Trial." NCBI. December 14, 2017. Accessed May 19, 2019. https://www.ncbi.nlm.nih.gov/pmc/articles/PMC5745680/.

Damle, S. G. "Smart Sugar? The Sugar Conspiracy." NCBI. July 24, 2017. Accessed March 7, 2019. https://www.ncbi.nlm.nih.gov/pmc/articles/PMC5551319/.

Dewan, Shalini Shahani. "Global Markets for Sugars and Sweeteners in Processed Foods and Beverages." Global Sugars and Sweeteners Market: Size, Share & Industry Report. BCC Research, 2015. https://www.bccresearch.com/market-research/food-and-beverage/sugar-sweeteners-processed-food-beverages -global-markets-report.html.

"Diet Review: Ketogenic Diet for Weight Loss." The Nutrition Source, May 22, 2019. https://www.hsph .harvard.edu/nutritionsource/healthy -weight/diet-reviews/ketogenic-diet/.

Feskanich et al., "Milk, dietary calcium, and bone fractures in women: a 12-year prospective study.," NCBI, June 1997, accessed September 11, 2017, https://www.ncbi.nlm.nih.gov/pmc/articles/PMC1380936/.

Finucane, O. M. et al.; "Monounsaturated Fatty Acid-Enriched High-Fat Diets Impede Adipose NLRP3 Inflammasome-Mediated IL-1β Secretion and Insulin Resistance despite Obesity," June 2015, https: //pubmed.ncbi.nlm.nih.gov/25626736/.

Garg, A.; "High-Monounsaturated-Fat Diets for Patients with Diabetes Mellitus: A Meta-Analysis," March 1998, https://pubmed.ncbi.nlm.nih .gov/9497173/.

Gearing, M., and S. McArdel, "Natural and Added Sugars: Two Sides of the Same Coin," October 5, 2015. https://sitn.hms.harvard.edu/flash /2015/natural-and-added-sugars-two-sides-of-the-same-coin/References263.

Gostin, Lawrence O. ""Big Food" Is Making America Sick." NCBI. September 13, 2013. Accessed March 7, 2019. https://www.ncbi.nlm.nih .gov/pmc/articles/PMC5020160/

"Hormones in Dairy Foods and Their Impact on Public Health—A Narrative Review Article," June 2015, accessed September 10, 2017, https://www.ncbi.nlm.nih.gov/pmc/articles /PMC4524299/.

Kaats, G. R., D. Bagchi, and H. G. Preuss. "Konjac Glucomannan Dietary Supplementation Causes Significant Fat Loss in Compliant Overweight Adults." NCBI. October 22, 2015. Accessed May 20, 2019. https: //www.ncbi.nlm.nih.gov/pubmed/26492494.

Kabara, J., D. Swieczkowski, A. Conley, and J. Truant. "Fatty Acids and Derivatives as Antimicrobial Agents." NCBI. July 1972. Accessed May 19, 2019. https://www.ncbi.nlm.nih.gov/pmc/articles/PMC444260/.

Koller, V. J., M. Furhacker, A. Nersesyan, M. Misik, M. Eisenbauer, and S. Knasmueller. "Cytotoxic and DNA-damaging Properties of Glyphosate and Roundup in Human-Derived Buccal Epithelial Cells." NCBI. May 2012. Accessed May 11, 2019. https://www.ncbi.nlm.nih.gov/pubmed/22331240.

Malekinejad, A., and H. Rezabakhsh. "Hormones in Dairy Foods and Their Impact on Public Health—A Narrative Review Article." *Iranian Journal of Public Health.* U.S. National Library of Medicine, June 2015. https://pubmed.ncbi.nlm.nih.gov/26258087/.

Maruyama, Kazumi, T. Oshima, and K. Ohyama, "Exposure to exogenous estrogen through intake of commercial milk produced from pregnant cows.," NCBI, February 2010, accessed September 20, 2017, https://pubmed.ncbi.nlm.nih.gov/19496976/.

McNamara, Donald. "The Fifty Year Rehabilitation of the Egg." NCBI. October 2015. Accessed April 27, 2019. https://www.ncbi.nlm.nih.gov/pmc/articles/PMC4632449/.

Michaëlsson, K. et al., "Milk intake and risk of mortality and fractures in women and men: cohort studies.," NCBI, October 28, 2014, accessed September 20, 2017, https://www.ncbi.nlm.nih.gov/pubmed/25352269.

Missimer, A., D. DiMarco, C. Andersen, A. Murillo, M. Vergara-Jiminez, and M. Fernandez. "Consuming Two Eggs per Day, as Compared to an Oatmeal Breakfast, Decreases Plasma Ghrelin While Maintaining the LDL/HDL Ratio." NCBI. February 01, 2017. Accessed April 27, 2019. https://www.ncbi.nlm.nih.gov /pmc/articles/PMC5331520/.

Mozaffarian, Dariush, Tao Hao, Eric Rimm, Walter Willett, and Frank Hu. "Changes in Diet and Lifestyle and Long-Term Weight Gain in Women and Men." *New England Journal of Medicine.* June 29, 2011. Accessed April 14, 2019. https://www.nejm.org/doi/full/10.1056 /NEJMoa1014296.

Mumme, K., and W. Stonehouse. "Effects of Medium-chain Triglycerides on Weight Loss and Body Composition: A Meta-Analysis of Randomized

Controlled Trials." NCBI. February 2015. Accessed May 19, 2019. https://www.ncbi.nlm.nih.gov/pubmed/25636220.

Nestle, M. "Food Lobbies, the Food Pyramid, and U.S. Nutrition Policy." NCBI. July 1, 1993. Accessed February 16, 2019. https://www.ncbi.nlm.nih.gov/pubmed/8375951.264

Ng, S. W., M. M. Slining, and B. M. Popkin. (2012). Use of caloric and noncaloric sweeteners in US consumer packaged foods, 2005–2009. *Journal of the Academy of Nutrition and Dietetics* 112(11), 1828–1834.

Niaz, K., E. Zaplatic, and J. Spoor. "Extensive Use of Monosodium Glutamate: A Threat to Public Health?" NCBI. March 19, 2018. Accessed May 11, 2019. https://www.ncbi.nlm.nih.gov/pmc/articles/PMC5938543/.

Paoli, Antonio. "Ketogenic Diet for Obesity: Friend or Foe?" NCBI. February 01, 2014. Accessed March 23, 2019. https://www.ncbi.nlm.nih.gov/pmc/articles/PMC3945587/.

C. S. Pase et al., "Influence of perinatal trans fat on behavioral responses and brain oxidative status of adolescent rats acutely exposed to stress," NCBI, September 05, 2013, accessed September 02, 2017, https: //www.ncbi.nlm.nih.gov/pubmed/23742847.

Samsel, A., and S. Seneff. "Glyphosate, Pathways to Modern Diseases II: Celiac Sprue and Gluten Intolerance." NCBI. December 2013. Accessed May 11, 2019. https://www.ncbi.nlm.nih.gov/pmc/articles/PMC3945755/.

Santarelli, R. L., F. Pierre, and D. Corpet. "Processed Meat and Colorectal Cancer: A Review of Epidemiologic and Experimental Evidence." NCBI. March 25, 2008. Accessed April 14, 2019. https://www.ncbi.nlm.nih.gov/pmc/articles/PMC2661797/.

Spero, David. "Is Milk Bad for You? Diabetes and Milk." Diabetes Self Management, June 20, 2017. https://www.diabetesselfmanagement.com/blog/is-milk-bad-for-you -diabetes-and-milk/.

"Sugar & The Diet." The Sugar Association. Accessed March 5, 2020. https://www.sugar.org/diet/.

Zhang, G., A. Pan, G. Zhong, Z. Yu, H. Wu, X. Chen, L. Tang, Y. Feng, H. Zhou, H. Li, B. Hong, W. C. Willett, V. S. Malik, D. Spiegelman, F. B. Hu, and X. Lin. "Substituting White Rice with Brown Rice for 16 Weeks Does Not Substantially Affect Metabolic Risk Factors in Middle-Aged Chinese Men and Women with Diabetes or a High Risk for Diabetes." NCBI. September 01, 2011. Accessed April 14, 2019. https://pubmed.ncbi.nlm.nih.gov/21795429/.

Tribute to
Dr. Val Manocchio

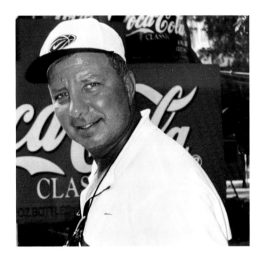

With twenty-two years in practice as an anesthesiologist, Dr. Val Manocchio had focused his career on medical weight for more than a decade. When blood clots in his lungs during surgery left him bedridden for over a year, this wake-up call motivated him to study nutrition and fitness. With a new outlook on life, he lost fifty-five pounds using his own dietary products and supplements and opened Doctors Best Wellness Center in South Florida. Val said, "I can honestly say I save more lives today than I ever did in the operating room." This book pays tribute to the knowledge and expertise of Dr. Val Manocchio, who unfortunately passed away in 2020. He is remembered through his wife Rachael and two children, Nick and Alex.

About the Authors

Aimee Aristotelous, author of *Super Simple Keto*, *Almost Keto*, *The 30-Day Keto Plan*, and *The Whole Food Pregnancy Plan*, is a certified nutritionist, specializing in ketogenic and gluten-free nutrition, as well as prenatal dietetics. Aristotelous is a contributor for a variety of publications including *Health*, *People*, *HuffPost*, *Parade*, *Yahoo! News*, *INSIDER*, *Motherly*, *Consumer Health Digest*, *Simply Gluten-Free*, *Well + Good*, National Celiac Association, and Delight Gluten-Free. She has appeared on the morning show in Los Angeles, as a regular speaker for the nationwide Nourished Festival, and has been the exclusive nutritionist for NBC affiliate KSEE 24 News in California, appearing in more than fifty nutrition and cooking segments. Aimee has nine years of nutrition consulting experience and has helped over 3,000 people lose weight and get healthy!

Aimee's interest in nutrition began as she struggled with her own high cholesterol and weight gain after taking a sedentary office job in her twenties, once her athletic career came to an end. She furthered her nutrition education in the ketogenic and gluten-free realms after applying those dietary lifestyles to resolve her bad cholesterol, weight gain, and other dietary-related ailments such as migraine headaches. In addition to her Nutrition and Wellness certification through American Fitness Professionals and Associates, Aimee has a bachelor's degree in business/marketing from California State University, Long Beach. A California native, she currently resides in Fort Lauderdale, Florida, with her husband, Richard, and son, Alex, and enjoys the beach, cooking, and traveling.

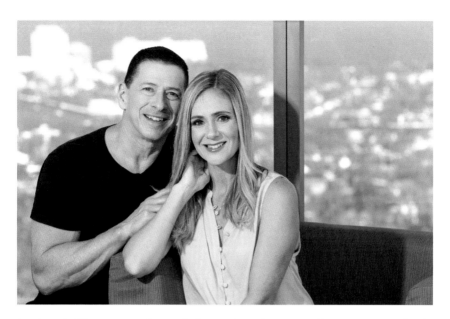

Richard Oliva, coauthor of *Super Simple Keto*, *Almost Keto*, and *The 30-Day Keto Plan*, is a certified nutritionist who specializes in ketogenic, gluten-free, and sports nutrition. He is a third-degree black belt in judo who has competed internationally and won state, national, and international titles. Oliva has conducted numerous nutrition seminars for colleges, health clubs, and medical practices, and has appeared in numerous nutrition and cooking segments on NBC affiliate KSEE 24 News in California. He loves to share his lifetime passion for both nutrition and judo and has helped thousands of people learn how to eat better and improve their health and fitness.

Richard began studying nutrition at about the same time that he started learning judo in the mid-1970s, when he was in high school. He became a passionate student of nutrition after one of his coworkers told him, "You know, you're killing yourself!" as Richard was eating a donut and drinking a soda during his break. That comment launched him on a mission to learn everything he could about nutrition and health.

Richard earned his Nutrition and Wellness certification through American Fitness Professionals and Associates. He also has a Bachelor of Science degree in geology from Kent State University in Kent, Ohio. An

Ohio native, he currently resides in Fort Lauderdale, Florida, with Aimee and Alex. Richard still enjoys practicing judo as well as weight training, cooking, and traveling.

Founder and CEO of Doctors Weight Loss, **Christian Forster** has been involved in the health and wellness industry for twenty years, and is passionate about improving the lives of his customers, team members, and their families. Inspired by his brother-in-law and business partner, Val 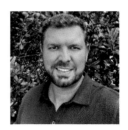 Manocchio, MD, Doctors Weight Loss began as a small weight loss clinic in 2008. It quickly gained a following due to the program's success rate, and not long after, its three flagship brands, NutriWise, Protiwise, and BestMed Weight Loss were developed. They are committed to ensuring top-quality formulations while customers are able to pay only a fraction of the high prices offered at most competing weight loss clinics.

After establishing two successful locations in Florida, Doctors Weight Loss decided to take the clinic model online to bring the same effective weight loss products to customers nationwide. The Doctors Weight Loss Diet helps customers understand and implement the high-protein, low-carbohydrate protocol, with the optional convenience of meal plans which incorporate pre-packed medical-grade weight loss products that truly "taste like you're cheating." Born and raised in Nottingham, England, Christian currently lives between Miami and North Carolina, and enjoys playing tennis, traveling, and spending time with his wife, Shannon, and children, Connor, Ryan, Madison, and Max.

Dr. Katherine Rodriguez was born and raised in Miami. She completed Commissioned Officer Training at Maxwell Air Force Base in August, 2000, before beginning her first year at Albert Einstein College of Medicine. Her love of metropolitan culture led her to spend her summers in Paris, her medical training in New York, and business expansion in Dubai. Now back in south Florida, she continues her medical career aspiring to prevent diseases that can lead patients to the hospital.

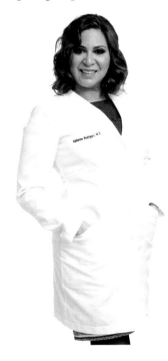

Out-of-control weight has long clouded happiness in many people's lives. Once a patient makes that decision to take control of their health, then their destiny is also in their own hands. A hospital is no place for a healthy person and so Dr. Rodriguez has dedicated her medical practice to functional medicine, treating patients with modern medical therapies, including RegenerWave, a low-intensity extracorporal shockwave therapy that causes neoangiogenesis for pain and inflammation. Immunomodulation is key to age repair. Reaching and maintaining an ideal weight will enhance longevity and vitality.

Conversion Charts

Metric and Imperial Conversions

(These conversions are rounded for convenience)

Ingredient	Cups/Tablespoons/ Teaspoons	Ounces	Grams/Milliliters
Butter	1 cup/ 16 tablespoons/ 2 sticks	8 ounces	230 grams
Cheese, shredded	1 cup	4 ounces	110 grams
Cream cheese	1 tablespoon	0.5 ounce	14.5 grams
Fruit, dried	1 cup	4 ounces	120 grams
Fruits or veggies, chopped	1 cup	5 to 7 ounces	145 to 200 grams
Fruits or veggies, pureed	1 cup	8.5 ounces	245 grams
Liquids: cream, milk, water, or juice	1 cup	8 fluid ounces	240 milliliters
Salt	1 teaspoon	0.2 ounce	6 grams
Spices: cinnamon, cloves, ginger, or nutmeg (ground)	1 teaspoon	0.2 ounce	5 milliliters
Vanilla extract	1 teaspoon	0.2 ounce	4 grams

Oven Temperatures

Fahrenheit	Celsius	Gas Mark
225°	110°	¼
250°	120°	½
275°	140°	1
300°	150°	2
325°	160°	3
350°	180°	4
375°	190°	5
400°	200°	6
425°	220°	7
450°	230°	8

Index

Also Available

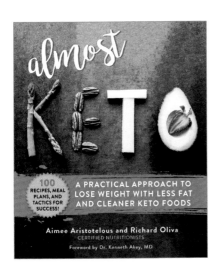

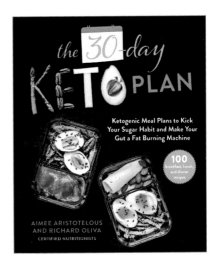

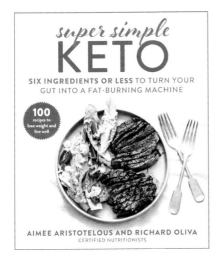

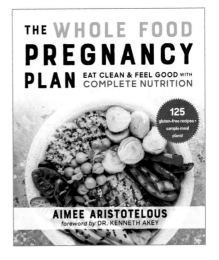